Impaired Driving Shattered Lives

Robert L. Bryan

Impaired Driving

Shattered Lives

By Robert L. Bryan

Copyright 2018   by Robert L. Bryan

2018 New York

For Meghan

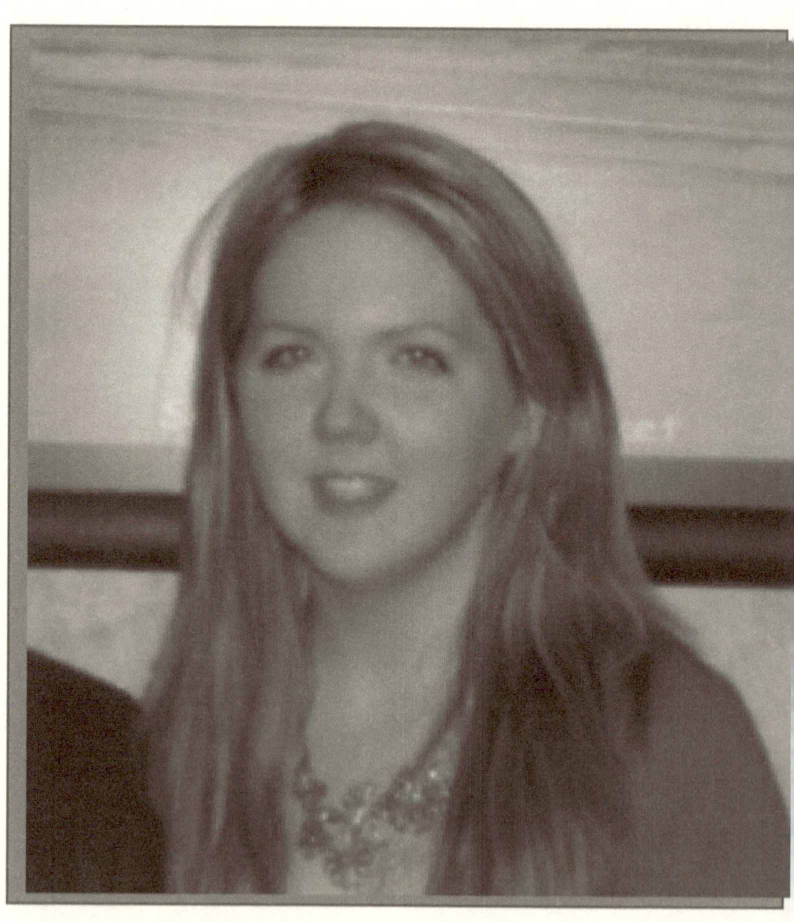

Contents

Forward

Less than a week after a gunman killed 14 students and three staff at Marjory Stoneman Douglas High School in Parkland, Florida, survivors of the shooting mobilized to launch the #NeverAgain movement, and the March for Our Lives, a nationwide protest against gun violence.

"Not one more," the organization's mission statement reads. "We cannot allow one more child to be shot at school. We cannot allow one more teacher to make a choice to jump in front of a firing assault rifle to save the lives of students. We cannot allow one more family to wait for a call or text that never comes. Our schools are unsafe. Our children and teachers are dying. We must make it our top priority to save these lives."

My heart goes out to those who lost loved ones in this horrendous attack. This school shooting, along with all the other terrible active shooter incidents, merit the full attention of the public and our government officials so that necessary steps can be taken to prevent any further acts of violence. When parents send a child to school, they should be secure in the knowledge that their child is in a safe environment. Parents have every right to know what schools are doing to protect their children from an active shooter event.   The organizers of the #NeverAgain movement should be applauded for raising the consciousness of the nation. But let's momentarily hit the pause button of our outrage to consider some additional facts. Parents also have the right to information regarding all the threats to their children. As horrible as the image of an active shooter in a school may, most parents would be surprised to learn that statistically, their children face a far greater threat.   In 2015 twenty victims of shootings in United States schools were killed. Contrast that statistic with the fact that of the 10,265 people killed in the United States in 2015 in alcohol-impaired driving crashes, 209 of the victims were children (NHTSA)

A school age child is ten times more likely to be killed by an impaired driver than in a school shooting. That statistic should be enough to get every parent's attention regarding the extent of the problem of impaired driving.

Sunday afternoon, December 18, 2011, at approximately 4:00PM, my plan was coming together perfectly. I was making my closing remarks to thirty students in a defensive driving class at the Italian Charities Hall in the Elmhurst section of Queens, New York City. I officially concluded the class and said my goodbyes to the students as I collected their course evaluation sheets. Finally, the last student exited through the classroom door and I was alone. Eureka! I had made it through the entire afternoon without one student making reference to the score of the Giants / Redskins football game. I was recording the game at home, and all I had to do now was drive home without the radio on and I could enjoy the game as if I were watching it live. Finally, one of my plans was actually going to work. I gathered up my classroom materials and headed towards my car that was parked in a meter on Queens

Blvd. Sunday classes at the Italian Charities Hall were palatable

because parking meter regulations were lifted on Sunday's, so I

could park all day in the meter directly in front of the hall. I

placed my box of materials on the roof of my 2011 Kia Rio and

searched my pants pockets for my keys. My search was

interrupted before completion by the vibration of my cell phone.

It was my daughter Meghan calling from her boyfriend's house.

"Hi daddy-boy." Meghan sang out using her standard nickname

for me. "What's up Meg?" I countered while continuing my key

search with my free hand. Meghan continued, "How could the

Giants have been so awful daddy-boy?" I momentarily suspended

my key search and stood with the phone to my left ear and my

mouth wide open in utter disbelief. My plan had just been

completely shattered by my own daughter. I probably should

have realized the danger to my plan when her call came in right as

the game was likely to be ending. More significant was the fact that Meghan's boyfriend was a big Giants fan, and Meghan was starting to take an interest in football and the Giants. I watched parts of several games with her that season, and I still remember how funny she found it when Giants wide receiver Victor Cruz would score a touchdown and break into his patented Salsa dance. Oh well, as Robert Burns noted, "The best laid plans of mice and men often go awry."

Monday morning, December 19, 2011 was nothing more than routine. During this time period I worked on Saturdays and my days off were Sunday and Monday. My usual Monday routine called for me to drive Meghan and Bryan to school. Meghan was a senior at Molloy College in nearby Rockville Centre, and Bryan was finishing up his first freshman semester at Molloy. The only non-routine aspect to the morning was the fact that Meghan was taking a final in one of her major subjects – speech pathology. Meghan was not a naturally gifted student, but she was relentless with her studies and had received very good grades during her college years. I could tell that this particular examination had her on edge. As she went about her morning routine, she never let go of a stack of index cards containing the subject material for the test. It was also clear to me that the pace of the household was progressing too slowly to suit Meghan. Her exam was at 10 AM and it took approximately 20-30 minutes to drive from Bellerose to Molloy. Now, as the clock moved past 9 AM, Bryan was not even in the shower yet and breakfast had not been served. With Meghan becoming increasingly more nervous regarding the time, I made a decision. Meghan's final was at 10 AM, but Bryan's first class did not begin until 11 AM. I decided to leave with Meghan immediately – drop her off in time for the final – then come back and get Bryan to Molloy in time for his class. Meghan loved the idea and within five minutes we were on our way. We had not eaten breakfast so I stopped at the drive thru window of a nearby Burger King and ordered breakfast for Meghan. For the remainder of the trip, I don't remember any specific conversations we had. I recall not wanting to bother Meghan as she studied her

index cards, and I'm sure I must have asked her what time she

expected to be finished with the exam. Again, everything about

the drive to school was routine. I drove this route many times

before over the past 3.5 years, and at approximately 9:30 AM I

was on the last leg of the trip. My usual route placed me

southbound on Peninsula Boulevard in the Village of Hempstead.

I would make a left turn onto West Marshall Street, drive through

a residential neighborhood before making a right turn on South

Franklin Street, and almost immediately thereafter entering the

main gate of Molloy College.

I recall accessing the left turn lane on Peninsula Boulevard in

anticipation of my left onto West Marshall. The traffic signal was

green, but northbound traffic prohibited me from turning across

the three lanes of traffic – so I waited in the intersection. The light

turned red and northbound traffic on peninsula came to a stop,

allowing me to complete my left turn.

The best way I can articulate what followed is to describe the events as a series of still photographs. From my perception, my memories became like a photo album, filled with still images.

My first memory was of a very loud "popping" sound, combined with a "bounce" of the car as if it had been lifted a few feet by the front fender and then dropped. What happened next is still very hard to describe. I recall that my environment was very quiet. I was aware something had just happened, but I could not wrap my brain around what might have just transpired. I recall staring at the dashboard and noting the deflated airbag, but still not being able to figure out what had happened. I could see everything inside the car, but it was as if the interior of the car was where my world ended, as I could not see anything going on outside. I was sitting back in the driver's seat and Meghan was leaning forward with her head appearing to be resting on the dashboard. I do not recall seeing any blood or obvious signs of injury from Meghan or myself. The next observation I recall making was recognizing that

I was no longer wearing my eyeglasses and trying to understand what had happened to them. Meghan never moved or spoke as reality began to take shape in my brain. I was not in any pain at this time, and although I do not recall trying to get out of my seat, I knew that I was unable to move – if that makes any sense. I recall vividly reaching out with my right hand and rubbing Meghan's back, while commenting as a statement to her and a question to myself, "I think we got hit, Meg." I kept rubbing her back and telling her that everything would be alright. It was at that moment that the thought entered my brain that the situation was bad – very bad. My sense of time was completely gone, so I have no idea how much time had passed when I began to hear voices and activity from what seemed like all around me. My visual world was still limited to the dashboard and Meghan, and I could not see any rescue personnel. I recall many voices and a lot of shouting from all around. I felt a hand on my shoulder and a voice ask my name. Anytime I perceived someone was addressing me I would respond by saying "Please help my daughter." I have no memories of anyone moving or working on Meghan, but I know I heard a voice say "She's responding", which providing me a glimmer of hope. As I progress through my album of still images I recall sparks and the sound of a loud machine. Later, I learned that I had to be cut out of the driver's seat. When I was able to be extricated from the car, my world quickly transitioned from no pain to the most intense pain I had ever experienced. From that moment forward, I have very few memories because the only factor consuming my brain was the intense pain. Obviously, there was no room to store any other images or memories. I recall being in a bed with numerous doctors and nurses who seemed to be moving all around me. It seemed as if every minute a different nurse would ask me my name, my date of birth, my address, and if I knew where I was. They were also constantly asking my pain level on a scale of one to ten, to which I would always respond "one hundred." I recall a doctor saying "Give him morphine," followed by the weirdest feeling as the pain completely subsided body part by body part as the morphine made its way through me. Without the pain to consume me, I asked the next nurse who approached my bed, "What happened?" She said, "You were in a car accident." I followed up with "Where is my daughter?" but she walked away from the bed without answering. Her lack of response spoke volumes. At some point a woman approached my bed. This woman was not dressed in the typical doctor / nurse attire. I don't remember her name or what she looked like, but I do recall that she introduced herself as the hospital administrator. Her message was brief and to the point. Meghan's injuries were too severe and she had passed away. I did not respond. The administrator had been on the right side of my bed, and I recall focusing on a light fixture that was on the ceiling past my feet on the left side of the bed. I just stared at the fixture. My body and my brain were numb.

I still had no concept of how much time had passed, but I recall a priest anointing me. With the morphine in full effect, I was in no pain, and I remember thinking with a tinge of amusement "Wow, I must really be in bad shape." But at that point, I really didn't care.

Familiar faces began to join the legions of doctors and nurses. It's difficult to remember the order of appearances, but I do recall that my mother-in-law and sister-in-law were the first familiar faces I recognized at my bedside. Eventually, I recall my wife and son appearing. For all I went through, I still don't know how they were able to hold things together during this horrendous time. Meghan had been transported to a different hospital, and as unbelievable as this might seem, they were given the name of the wrong hospital for Meghan's location. I can't begin to imagine the stress, grief and frustration they experienced that day. As for me, I sustained a broken neck, broken back, all my ribs were broken, my right hand was broken, and most of my teeth were knocked out. Additionally, I sustained damage to my perneal nerve that still requires me to where a brace on my lower left leg and foot. I was lucky. It took several months, but aside from the brace on my leg, everything healed and my normal life functions continued. Meghan was gone.

I don't remember who first told me what had happened. It may have been my wife or another relative or it may have been a police detective. At some point, however during either the 19th or 20th I was told the story. An impaired driver high on cocaine, driving at a high rate of speed north on Peninsula Boulevard, had drove through the red signal and T-boned my vehicle directly on the passenger side door. To this day I have no recollection of the other vehicle or the impact – just that "popping" sound.

The worst part of the weeks in the hospital and rehabilitation facility was the time alone – thinking. If anything almost broke me it was these times where I would lay there for hours on end thinking about how I got to that intersection at the exact moment that the other car ran the red light. What if we didn't stop at

Burger King? What if I waited a few minutes for Bryan to get ready? What if Meghan forgot something and had to go back into the house to get it? What if I drove slightly faster or slower? It seemed that any slight alteration would have prevented me from being in that intersection at that precise moment. I was literally driving myself crazy. On Christmas Eve I lay alone in the hospital while Meghan was buried.

When I finally returned home was when reality really set in. Meghan was not there and would never be there. For awhile I was still not able to navigate the stairs in the house. When I finally could climb the stairs I visited Meghan's room. Everything was as it was on the morning of December 19th. I could still actually smell her in the room. It was too much to bear, and it was many, many months before I returned to her room.

As the years roll by, I knew the holidays would be tough periods, but I soon learned that everyday life was just as tough. Almost every day, some innocuous place or incident reminds me of

Meghan. Every time I watch the Giants on TV, I am reminded of her delight at watching the touchdown dance. When I drive past St. Gregory's, her grammar school, I can see her smiling face walking towards me as if I were once again picking her up after school. Not a day goes by that I don't think of her. Sometimes it makes me feel good and sometimes it doesn't. While I was hospitalized I was visited by several different Chaplains. I am retired from the New York City Police Department and currently work for the New York City Transit Authority, so I was visited by Chaplains from the NYPD, the TA, as well as a Chaplain from the hospital. One of these Chaplains said something that stayed with me. He said that the grief of losing Meghan will remain with me forever, but that the deep grief will subside. I did not understand what he meant then, but I do now. The deep depression and grief I experienced in the initial weeks after Meghan's death could not be sustained. I would not have been able to function with that frame of mind. So eventually, the grief did lessen and I was able to go on with life. A life, however, that was forever changed by a

selfish man who made the choice to get high on cocaine and then

get behind the wheel with a suspended license and drive at a high

rate of speed, through a red light, and kill my daughter. That is

the face of impaired driving

Introduction

Is my story unique? Were Meghan and I simply victimized by being in the wrong place at the wrong time, akin to being struck by a tiny fragment of a meteor that was able to pass into the earth's atmosphere? Unfortunately, my story is far from unique

Imagine a collection of high school students standing vigil in an open field. At their feet is a gold and black football helmet, a variety of wildflowers, and the photograph of a friend who'd died not long before when his car was struck by a drunk driver. These were the friends of one Michael Finley of Falcon, Colorado. Finley, 18, was a model student, football star, and member of the student council. One day, he hoped to become a police officer. The man who struck him was arrested and, at the time of this writing, is being held under suspicion of drunk driving and vehicular homicide.

Now imagine an 18-year old girl is texting and updating her Facebook status behind the wheel of her pickup truck. Her friend is pleading with her to put the phone away. Instead, she insists on continuing until she runs through a red light, striking a passing mini-van and killing a man and his 10-year old daughter. Carlee Bollig plead guilty to two counts of criminal vehicular homicide after the July crash that claimed the life of 54-year-old Charles Maurer and his daughter Cassey.

These stories, though tragic, are not remarkable. In 2015, 10,265 people died in crashes related to drunk driving. That's roughly one death every 50 minutes or 28 deaths a day. That's a dramatic increase from the 9,967 drunk driving deaths reported in 2014, suggesting that despite painful stories like Finley's, people just aren't taking the matter seriously.

As for texting and driving, the Department of Transportation reported 3,154 deaths and 424,000 injuries in 2013 as a result of cell phone use in the car. Despite many states taking steps to ban this behavior, Americans don't seem to be getting the message. A survey conducted by AT&T quizzed adults on their cell phone habits when behind the wheel of a car. More than a quarter of those adults admitted to sending or reading text messages while their vehicle was in motion.

Impaired driving, be it from substance use, exhaustion, distraction, or something else is a serious matter. Say that to any random person on the street and they're sure to agree with you. Then how come there are still so many accidents? Why do people still get behind the wheel of a car when they feel even slightly buzzed? Why do they reach for their cell phones when they know in their hearts that the text they are about to send is not as important as the lives they're putting at risk?

This book seeks to explore the phenomenon of impaired driving. We will discuss all forms of impaired driving from drunk driving to road rage. We'll tackle the statistics to better understand the impact these acts have on our community and look to case studies to put faces on those numbers. By thoroughly tackling the reality and consequences of these acts, we can better look to solutions. If you take nothing else away from this book, let it be that you think

twice the next time you want to drive home after a night out or

pull out your cell phone when you should be watching the road.

Impaired Definition: Weakened or damaged.

We're going to be saying "impaired driving" quite a bit, so we should be clear about what we mean when we use this term. In truth, there is some inconsistency in how this term is defined, making it difficult to appreciate what stats associated with impaired driving really mean.

For example, the Foundation for Traffic Safety uses "impaired driving" to refer to any driving done under the influence of a physical substance, be it alcohol, illicit drugs, or even prescribed medications. The legal acronym DWI (Driving While Intoxicated) similarly refers only to the use of alcohol. However, the Center for Disease Control (CDC) and the National Highway Traffic Safety Administration (NHTSA) discern between alcohol-impaired driving and other forms of impaired driving. The NHTSA lists distracted driving and drowsy driving as risky driving behaviors alongside alcohol-impaired driving.

Confused yet? Don't worry. All you really need to understand is that it's complicated and that you'll want to be clear about how an organization defines impaired driving when you look at their statistics. We've made it even simpler and looked to the definition of impaired to inform our approach to "impaired driving."

As noted in the beginning of this chapter, impaired means "weakened or damaged." If your driving is impaired, then it has been weakened. What weakens driving?

- Alcohol
- Illicit drugs use
- Legal drug use
- Exhaustion
- Medical conditions
- Distraction from technology
- Distraction from environmental factors
- Road rage

When we talk about impaired-driving, we'll be referring to any of the impairments listed above.

For now, let's take some time to introduce each of these types of impaired driving and how they weaken one's ability to operate a motor vehicle.

Alcohol (or Drunk Driving)

This one is fairly straight-forward. You've likely already heard all about it in half a dozen high school assemblies. It is illegal in all states to drive while intoxicated and in most states to even have an open container of alcohol in the car. In our chapter on drunk driving, we'll take a closer look at what it means to be intoxicated, the consequences of drunk driving, and methods for preventing it. We will also try very hard to avoid the semblance of "Preaching". Let's be clear – the purpose of this book is not to point out the evils of drinking alcohol, but simply to point out how alcohol effects the body, and how those effects are negative when we translate them into the skills necessary to safely drive. Alcohol quickly erodes a person's judgement, reflexes, and vision – all critical skills necessary to safely drive. As we delve into the topic of drinking and driving, please think of the issue figuratively like a slope, instead of a cliff. What does this mean? At some point in this book we will discuss legal limits as it relates to drinking and driving. But you should not think of the issue like a cliff, where you may had had a drink or two and then "Wham", just like going over a cliff you have the drink that puts you over the legal limit and everything about your driving goes bad. Instead, you should think of the issue like a slope. Beginning with your first drink you are on a downward slope and your skills are eroding. At some point on that slope you will pass a legal limit, but it's not just drinking when you have reached a legal limit that is a problem – any drinking will have a negative impact on your ability to safely drive.

<u>Illicit Drug Use</u>

Drugs are a complicated matter not only because they come in legal and illegal forms, but also because even legal drugs can be used illegally. When we talk about illicit drug use, we're talking about illegal drugs (like cocaine or heroin), legal prescription drugs to which the driver does not have legal access (like Oxycontin or Vicodin), and legal over-the-counter drugs that are being abused (like cough syrup). In short, the "illicit" refers to the drug use and not necessarily the drug. We'll dig deeper into these distinctions and the legal ramifications of each in our chapter on drug use and related medical conditions.

<u>Legal Drug Use</u>

This category is far more innocent than the last in that it assumes little to no reckless behavior on the part of the driver. However, legal drugs that are used in prescribed or recommended amounts by the correct party can still impact driving, and anything that impacts driving can have dire consequences. This category typically refers to severe side effects or drug interactions that impact driving. In some cases, these effects may be rare or unexpected, absolving the driver of some responsibility. In other cases, it may be that the driver was not supposed to be operating a vehicle on the medication and chose to do so anyway, leaving them open to consequences. We'll explore these distinctions more in our chapter on drug use and related medical conditions.

<u>Exhaustion</u>

You could have nothing in your system. You could be an otherwise model citizen. But if you drive fatigued and nod off at the wheel, then you could be putting lives in danger. It's often considered the individual's legal responsibility to not operate a vehicle if they feel too tired to do so. Choosing to do otherwise may have legal ramifications. In our chapter on exhausted driving, we'll explore the importance of a good night's sleep and methods for staying awake. And consider one more factor. Of course the danger of falling asleep behind the wheel is a primary concern, but did you realize that when you are overly tired behind the wheel, you exhibit the exact same symptoms as if you were intoxicated.

<u>Medical Conditions</u>

This category is dedicated to those physical limitations that are not a result of substance use, exhaustion, or distraction. In some cases, medical conditions may be ongoing and well-known to the individual, but an attack could be unexpected (as with diabetes or asthma). In other cases, the entire condition may be unexpected (as with a heart attack or seizure). Typically, individuals who get into accidents because of a medical condition will not be held legally responsible unless they neglected to treat the condition or drove when they weren't supposed to. In our chapter on drug use and related medical conditions, we'll look more closely at the types of conditions that might arise, warning signs for strokes and asthma attacks, and methods for seeking help.

Distraction from Technology

While "texting while driving" is the most publicized and reviled form of distraction from technology while driving, it's hardly the only one. This category also includes the use of cell phones to interact with social media, look up directions on a map, or even make a phone call. In rare cases, drivers have even been reported using tablets and laptops while behind the wheel. We'll explore the incessant lure of technology and its effect on driving safety in our chapter on distracted driving.

Distraction from Environmental Factors

No, we're not talking about the weather, although the weather can be its own brand of distraction. We're referring to environmental factors from within the car. In other words, your child kicking the back of your seat as hard as he can or your girlfriend playing with your hair and tickling you. Anything going on around you in the car that could be taking your attention away from where it most needs to be is a distraction. We'll talk more about these factors

and how to address them in our chapter on distracted driving.

Remember, you only have one hundred percent of anything, and

when you're behind the wheel one hundred percent of your focus

needs to be on one activity, and one activity only – driving.

<u>Road Rage</u>

You probably didn't expect this one. Sure, road rage causes deaths

each year. You've no doubt heard about furious drivers getting out

of their cars with weapons and fatally harming someone who'd cut

them off a moment ago. But what does that have to do with

impaired driving? Those people aren't driving when they act on

their aggression. The truth is, road rage can do more than make

you act out inappropriately; it can affect your ability to drive.

Individuals have been so distracted by their frustration and so

busy giving choice hand signals to the guy in the next lane that

they run stop signs or rear end the drivers in front of them. These

cases may be less dramatic than the aforementioned rage

incidents, but they are still dangers resulting from distracted driving.

As you read on, you'll learn more about each of these forms of impaired driving, including some telling statistics, some tragic stories and, most importantly, some handy strategies for staying safe on the road.

In 1980, Candace Lightner of Fair Oaks, California lost her 13-year old daughter Cari when she was struck by a drunk driver. The driver had recently been arrested for another DUI at the time of accident, but that didn't stop the local police from telling Candace that he would likely see very little punishment. Lightner took matters into her own hands and founded the most widely known nonprofit dedicated to raising awareness about drunk driving.

Mothers Against Drunk Driving (MADD) is alive and well nearly four decades later and continues to be committed to preventing drunk driving and seeking harsher punishments for offenders. Although the group has come under some criticism for being too bureaucratic, they've had a tangible impact on drunk driving laws and the availability of information and resources for the public.

Many of the laws that we'll talk about in this section are compliments of MADD and their hard work over the years, including lowering the legal blood-alcohol limit and pushing to make ignition interlock technology a requirement in 18 states.

MADD also provides victim services for those who survived

accidents related to drunk driving or lost loved ones, more of

which we'll discuss later in this chapter.

Drunk Driving Statistics

The following statistics will help you develop an appreciation for

the broad impact of drunk driving and the scope of the problem.

These statistics are compliments of the NHTSA with the

Department of Transportation, the Department of Justice and

more.

Traffic Deaths and Injuries

- Alcohol related crashes accounted for 31% (nearly a third)

  of all traffic death in the US in 2014.

Traffic Deaths Involving Children

- Of the 9,967 deaths in 2014, 1,070 (19%) were children aged 14 and younger. (NHTSA)

- Of the 1,070 children aged 14 and under who died in 2014, over half of them were in the same car as the impaired driver. (NHTSA)

- In 2015, 181 children aged 14 and under died in drunk driving related crashes. (NHTSA)

- Those 181 child deaths are a 83% decrease from the year before (2014). (NHTSA)

- Those 181 child deaths are roughly 1.7% of the total drunk driving related deaths in 2015. (NHTSA)

Arrests and Convictions

- Over 1.1 million drivers were arrested for driving under the influence of alcohol or drugs in 2014. (DOJ)

- That 1.1 million drivers pales in comparison to the 121 million self-reported episodes of drunk driving that occurred in 2014. (MMWR)

- Between 50% and 75% of convicted drunk drivers each year continue to drive after their license has been suspended. (TRC)

Drunk Drivers

- Drunk driving is highest among those aged 26 to 29. (SBMHSA)

- Roughly a third of drunk drivers arrested are repeat offenders. (NHTSA)

- Men are more likely than women to be driving in fatal accidents. 23% of men were drunk in crashes vs. 15% of women. (NHTSA)

<u>Understanding Drunkenness</u>

To better understand how alcohol can negatively affect your ability to drive, let's examine the changes your body goes through when under the influence. We'll take a close look at how brain chemistry specifically impacts one's ability to drive safely.

Alcohol gets absorbed into the bloodstream through the walls of the small intestine and the stomach. From there, it can get to the brain very quickly. It alters brain chemistry by changing the levels of neurotransmitters, those chemicals responsible for delivering messages throughout the body. More specifically, it increases the effects of inhibitory neurotransmitters (those responsible for decreasing or slowing electrical activity), throwing them out of balance with the excitatory neurotransmitters, which do the opposite. Even more specifically, alcohol acts on the following chemicals, causing dramatic changes in mood, behavior, and the ability to function.

- Alcohol **increases GABA**, an inhibitory neurotransmitter that is known to cause sluggish movement and speech. It's also the chemical you feel when alcohol makes you calm or seems to slow the world down around you.

- Alcohol **increases dopamine**. You've likely heard of this chemical before. It's the same pleasing chemical that gives runners the oft named "runner's high." Dopamine is responsible for a lot of the good feelings and subsequent recklessness associated with alcohol consumption.

- Alcohol **decreases glutamate**, an excitatory neurotransmitter that, like others of its kind, increases brain activity.

We can take away from this the fact that the brain is slowing down. Messages are not being sent and received as efficiently as they once were. What's more, the person under the influence is likely feeling pretty good about the whole thing. This dramatic change in brain chemistry typically manifests in the following ways:

- Slurred speech

- Blurred vision

- Slowed reaction time

- Poor short-term memory

- Decreased hand-eye coordination

It's a small wonder that being drunk makes it difficult to safely drive a car. If you woke up one morning and everything was blurry, you lacked the hand-eye coordination to get dressed without great difficulty, and you didn't know your spouse was tossing a towel your way before it was already on the floor, you'd probably phone it in for the day and tell your boss you can't drive. Why don't drunk drivers have the same instinct? Somewhere between the bar and the car that dopamine kicks in and reminds them that everything is great. They feel calm, collected, and capable. They aren't.

<u>Separating Myth from Fact</u>

To be clear, it is not illegal to have a drink and then drive, but remember the cliff / slope analogy. Even though you may not be legally drunk or impaired, any drinking will have a negative impact on your ability to drive. Your blood-alcohol concentration (BAC) must be above a certain threshold (something we'll be discussing in more depth shortly). Because there is a little room for interpretation when it comes to drunkenness, it's easy for people to convince themselves that they are not too drunk to drive or that something as simple as a cup of coffee will make all the difference. Allow us to disabuse you of some of these notions.

Myth 1: Alcohol is a stimulant.

The truth is quite the opposite. Alcohol is a depressant. Depressants slow down activity in the brain and, as we've just discussed, alcohol does exactly that. Many people just think it's a stimulant because it helps them have fun or feel social. But feeling emotionally or socially stimulated is not the same as having your brain activity stimulated.

Myth 2: Drinking coffee sobers me up.

Not in the least. Coffee is a stimulant and may help give you a little jolt of energy. That may even help you drive slightly better by making you somewhat more alert. But coffee does not reduce the level of alcohol in your blood. You are still as drunk as you were before that cup of joe and driving is still dangerous.

Myth 3: I'm bigger so it takes a lot to make me drunk.

Does size impact alcohol tolerance? Possibly. So too does biology, how much you ate that morning, how much sleep you got last night, and more. There are so many factors involved in determining your level of tolerance that it's irresponsible to assume any degree of tolerance on any given night.

Myth 4: Being tipsy makes me a safer driver because I am more cautious.

Big no. Maybe you realize you're too drunk to drive and you're nervous and alert for that reason. Maybe you drive slower and are hyper-aware of obeying traffic laws. Remember that you feel that way because you know you are too impaired to drive. What's more, no amount of careful driving will make it easier for your drunk eyes to see a stop sign coming up in the dark or your poor reaction time to hit the brakes when someone goes darting across the road.

Myth 5: You have to be driving to be charged with a DUI.

This one depends on the state. However, in many states, you can be arrested for a DUI just for being behind the wheel of a car, even if that car is off. Being behind the wheel suggests that you are taking control of the vehicle, and that's illegal. In other states, you can even be arrested after you've gotten out of car if it's clear that you were just operating it while drunk.

Next time you are debating driving yourself home from a bar and are trying to talk yourself into it with one of the above false claims, remember that your judgement is impaired thanks to alcohol. Let someone else make that decision for you.

All About Blood Alcohol Level

Let's revisit two key points that we made in the last section. First, BAC is responsible for determining if you are too drunk to drive. Second, drunkenness is a sliding scale, making it difficult for individuals to tell if they really are too drunk. We're going to take a closer look at the concept of blood-alcohol level and examine what it feels like to have your blood-alcohol level at certain points.

Let's set the scene. You're at your best friend's bachelor party. As best man, it's your duty to get the celebration going. In true best man form, you order a round of shots for you and your pals. This is going to be a good night.

BAC of .02%

It's been maybe thirty minutes since that shot and you're nursing a beer. You still feel very much ready to take on the night, but the shot definitely got your buzz started. Your inhibitions are lowered somewhat, enough that you don't mind checking out the bartender, but not so much that you're going to ask for her number. You're feeling relaxed and confident. A toasty warm feeling is creeping up from your toes and you're thinking about dancing. One of your buddies says something to you and you realize you haven't been paying attention.

BAC of .05%

It's been over a couple of hours now and the beers have kept coming regularly. You started dancing ten minutes ago. Too bad the people on the dance floor keep splitting in two as your vision blurs and occasionally doubles. You're eyeing the bartender again and start making your way over, playing through tacky pickup lines in your head. The bar seems further away than you thought and you trip over a stool on your way. You still feel like yourself though and you're able to pull it together enough to make her like you.

BAC of .08% - this is the legal limit

You have no idea how long it's been or how you landed yourself back on the dance floor. The bartender gave you her number and you're pretty sure you put it in your pocket, but you can't find it. She also gave you another shot. When you make your way back to where your buddies are sitting, they are cracking up at you. Apparently, your dance moves were less Michael Jackson and more Michael Meyers. One of your friends tells you they want to go back to their house for a bachelor after-party. You forget whose house before you're even outside of the bar.

BAC of .10% - this was the legal limit prior to 2000

You're in the parking lot, spending about ten minutes staring at a red fiesta that looks vaguely like your Prius, reading the word Fiesta over and over again and wondering if it's your car. You have to put a lot of concentration into keeping the letters from blurring beyond recognition. A friend puts his hand on your shoulder and guides you to your car. He asks if you feel ok to drive. You begin to tell him that you feel clear-headed enough to make it home, but you forget a few of the words you need to finish the sentence. He then reminds you that you're all going to an after-party. You nod and get in the car. When you turn it on and boost the headlights, the light on the pavement is hypnotizing, and you spend about five minutes just staring and letting your mind wander. Even though you have left the bar and are no longer drinking, your BAC continues to rise for a period of time until all the alcohol is absorbed into your blood stream.

BAC of .15%

You're driving. You are trying so hard not to go too fast that you are braking a little too hard every few seconds. What's more, you know you're supposed to keep the car between the lines, but the lines keep moving. You try to use the car in front of you as a guide, but get confused about which of the cars going in your direction is the one in front of you. You drift awkwardly into the left lane and side swipe the car in your blind spot. They swerve into oncoming traffic. You know you messed up but you don't know how to stop. You swerve to the side of the road, lucky to not have anyone on that side, and come to a hard stop halfway in a drainage ditch. You immediately fall when you get out of the car and throw up in the grass. You then lay down for a while, falling asleep before you have a chance to check on the other car.

BAC of .08% is the legal limit. That means that if you are given a breathalyzer test and your BAC is determined to be .08% exactly, you will be arrested and charged. However, as you can see from the tale above, you were likely feeling too tipsy to drive safely well before you reached .08%. It's also important to note that the above story is a guide based on generalizations. These levels may feel different to you based on your particular body chemistry. You should use your body as your guide to inform you about whether or not you can drive. Any amount of feeling inebriated is too much.

Alcohol Elimination

We've painted a vivid picture regarding how easy it is to rather quickly drink your way above a legal limit and face the legal and sometimes tragic consequences. A natural question at this point would be – "You've painted a picture with very broad strokes. Please tell me specifically how many drinks will get me to a legal limit?" Unfortunately, no specific answer to this query is possible.   There are just too many individual factors involved with how a person will react to alcohol.

- A person's weight is a factor on how he/she will react to alcohol consumption. A larger person has more blood to mix with the alcohol, lowering the concentration of the alcohol in the blood. This is why it is important to remember that BAC means blood alcohol CONCENTRATION – not CONTENT.

- Alcohol does not affect men and women equally. Research indicates that alcohol's effects on females tend to be stronger and last longer. This is because women produce a smaller amount of *alcohol dehydrogenase*, an enzyme that breaks down alcohol in the stomach. As a result, women reach a peak BAC about 20 percent higher than men do when consuming the same amount of alcohol.

- The stronger the alcohol content in the beverage consumed, the higher the BAC will rise, and the longer it will take for the alcohol to be eliminated from the body.

- A larger drink will contain more alcohol and result in a higher BAC as well as a longer elimination period.

- Food in the stomach does not absorb alcohol, but it might slow the rate at which alcohol is absorbed. All consumed alcohol will get into the blood eventually.

- The faster a person consumes alcohol, the more quickly BAC will reach its peak. Spreading out drinking over time will result in lower peak BAC. For example, the BAC would reach a higher level if a person had three drinks in one hour then if a person had one drink each hour for three hours.

To summarize, we can't say exactly how fast a person's BAC will rise or the exact rate at which alcohol will be eliminated from the body. There are just too many individual factors to consider. People may drink the same amount of a beverage, but the percentage of alcohol in the blood depends on the gender, body weight, strength of the drink, size of the drink, whether there is food in the stomach, and time spent drinking. There is one factor, however, that is certain. After drinking to the point of intoxication, you can eat food, drink black coffee, and take a cold shower, and you will be a well fed, wide awake, clean drunk – but you'll still be drunk! The ONLY way the alcohol leaves your body is through the natural elimination process, and that is a slow process. On average, it will take about 1.5 hours for a drink to be eliminated. Do the math. If you have indulged in a full night of consistent drinking, it will take many hours for that alcohol to be eliminated from your body.

The Legal Ramifications of the Breathalyzer

If you are pulled over under suspicion of drunk driving and the officer has a breathalyzer test available, he or she will administer it. The test measures the weight of alcohol in a small portion of your blood. Preliminary breathalyzer tests are not admissible in court. However, in most states, they give police officers probable cause to administer more reliable tests. They would next conduct blood or urine tests to more accurately measure blood alcohol levels. These are admissible in court.

You can technically refuse a breathalyzer test, but it isn't recommended. Refusing to be tested will not protect you from the law and you could still suffer a license suspension or jail time. True, you may avoid giving the officer the necessary probable cause to conduct further tests. However, if there is enough evidence at the scene (such as open containers), you may still receive a DUI or DWI charge. What's more, your refusal to take the test will likely be used in court as evidence against you. Furthermore, in many states there exists an "implied consent" law. In states with this type law, when a driver took his/her driver's license, they were, in effect, consenting to be tested for alcohol. Therefore, refusal of a breathalyzer can be a traffic infraction and can result in the suspension or revocation of the driver's license.

<u>What to Expect in a Field Sobriety Test</u>

If a police officer suspects a driver is under the influence of alcohol or drugs, he or she will conduct three tests that together are known as the Standardized Field Sobriety Test (SFST). These tests will be performed in conjunction with a breathalyzer if the device is available or alone if it is not. Like the breathalyzer, the field sobriety test is typically used to gain probable cause for further investigation into a DUI. Also like the breathalyzer, drivers have the right to refuse the field sobriety test. The consequences of doing so are not as dire as those of refusing a breathalyzer.

Have you ever seen police officers in the movies shinning flashlights in the eyes of suspected drunk drivers? They are likely conducted the first of these three tests. Horizontal gaze nystagmus (HGN) is an involuntary jerking of the eye-ball. It typically occurs when people look up and to the side. However, the jerking is more pronounced and happens more readily in those under the influence of alcohol. The **HGN test** checks for this reaction in those suspected of drunk driving.

You've almost certainly seen images of people trying to walk in a straight line at the behest of a police officer. The **walk-and-turn test** requires those suspected of drunk driving to do exactly that. They are required to take nine steps along a straight line, touching heel and toe with each step. The driver must then turn on one foot and walk another nine steps in the other direction, maintaining balance the entire time. The driver is not permitted to use his or her arms.

The final test is the **one-leg stand test**. During this test, the driver must stand on one leg with the other raised about six inches from the ground. While doing this, the driver must count in intervals of one starting with one thousand. The driver is typically expected to do this for about 30 seconds. However, the test may last longer. The police officer checks to make sure the driver isn't swaying or using arms to help with balance.

The Legal Ramifications of Drunk Driving

Charges for drunk driving vary dramatically. They can range from misdemeanors to felonies. Penalties can range from license revocation and fines to jail time. If you are caught driving under the influence, the charges and penalties that you are subject to will depend on a variety of factors, including your BAC, whether or not you got into an accident, whether or not there were any casualties, and whether or not you have any prior DUI or DWI convictions on your record.

Legal Terms

If you are convicted of drunk driving, you may not hear the terms DUI or DWI, although these are the most common. There are a variety of acronyms and other terms having to do with drunk driving and related offenses. Bear in mind that different states use different terminologies to describe offenses, but they all come down to offenses involving drinking and driving.

- **DUI** – Driving under the influence

- **DWI** – Driving while impaired

- **OWI** – Operating a vehicle while impaired

- **OVI** – Operating a vehicle under the influence

- **DWAI** – Driving while ability impaired

- **DWUI** – Driving while under the influence

- **Vehicular homicide** – This is when a driver of a car causes the death of another person in their or another vehicle using the car. This can be intentional or unintentional. However, the driver must be deemed responsible for the choices that led to the unintentional death.

- **Vehicular manslaughter** – This refers exclusively to the unintentional death of an individual at the hands of a driver. It is a lesser charge that is typically used to replace vehicular manslaughter in cases where the driver's poor choices were less egregious.

- **DUI School** – Many of those convicted of driving under the influence are instructed to intent DUI school, which could include instruction on the dangers of drunk driving and group therapy.

- **Conditional license** – A license that places limitations on when a driver is allowed to drive.

License Suspension

The license suspension is a very common penalty for DUIs. In fact, your license may get suspended even if you're not formally convicted of a DUI as long as a chemical test shows a BAC at or above the legal limit. The later suspension would come directly from your state's Department of Motor Vehicles (DMV). If you show a BAC of at least .08% and are convicted of a DUI, you may actually get two license suspensions, one from the DMV and another from the judge. Whether these add up or overlap depends on your state.

If your license is suspended, you can't operate a vehicle with it. However, as long as it hasn't expired, you can use your license as valid identification. In fact, nothing on the license will indicate that it has been suspended. Sometimes, individuals continue driving as normal without realizing that their license has been suspended at all. When this happens, those individuals can be arrested for driving without a valid license.

You know your license has been suspended when your local DMV sends a written notice to the address they have on file for the license, which should be your address. If you don't recall seeing a written notice and want to know if your license has been suspended, you can also call or go online to your DMV website.

License suspensions can last anywhere from a few months to a few years depending on the severity of the offense. During this time, individuals are not allowed to drive under any circumstances, including to get to and from work. This is not to be confused with a conditional license which only suspends driving under certain circumstances.

Fines / Fees

Drunk driving fines are wildly variable. They could be as little as $500 or as much as $2000. When you add legal fees to the mix, you could be looking at over 20 thousand dollars in fines and legal fees combined. These are just the costs you find on paper. Those convicted of drunk driving may face lost wages due to jail time or an inability to get to work as a result of their license suspension. Basically, drunk driving convictions are expensive.

Fines depend on a variety of factors, including the severity of the offense (how drunk you were, whether you damaged any public property, etc), how many prior offenses you have on record, and your particular district or state.

Jail Time

Although drunk driving is dangerous, a drunk driving conviction will not absolutely end in jail time. Whether or not you're sentenced to jail depends on those same factors that play into the size of your fine: the severity of the offense, how many priors you have, and any other rules or policies specific to your area. If you are given jail time, the amount of time can also widely vary. Typically, first time offenders will not receive jail time unless their actions are considered particularly egregious.

Ways You Can Prevent Drunk Driving

No amount of special initiatives or public demonstrations can prevent a single instance of drunk driving as effectively as an individual taking it upon him or herself to make the right choice. That means that the best way to prevent drunk driving is by having resources and strategies in place to keep yourself from doing something you'll regret. Often that means making certain resources available to yourself before going out on the town.

Designated Driver

The classic drunk driving solution is the designated driver. If you're out with a group and going someplace that can't easily be accessed without a car, designate a friend to stay sober and be the ride home. Designated drivers should not drink at all. Once drinking starts, so too does the slippery slope to wondering if you're sober enough to drive.

Easy Cab Access

Understandably, you may not have a friend that's willing to be the sober one out. In that case, you need another ride home. If you're nowhere near public transportation, be ready to take a cab. Prepare for this ahead of time. Know where the nearest cab stand is or have cab company numbers readily available in your phone. Take a cab there if need be or park someplace where you feel comfortable leaving your car overnight. In this era of "Uber-type" transportation alternatives, there really is no excuse for being unable to find suitable transportation other than getting behind the wheel yourself.

Public Transportation

You may not typically use it, especially if your city is more prone to buses than subways, but it's a valid method for getting around. Make sure you know the public route home (and the way to the nearest stop) before you go out.

Stay Close to Home

If you and your friends live in the same area, consider a house party instead. Friends can walk home or crash if need be. Not to mention, house parties come with other nice perks. Closing time is when you say it is and the drinks will likely be cheaper.

Of course, you may feel confident that you're in no danger of driving drunk. However, that doesn't mean your best friend at the bar is quite as responsible. There are things you can do to help prevent others from driving drunk as well.

Volunteer

Your group needs a designated driver? You could always be that important person. Sure, it may seem like less fun. But there's more to going out than just getting drunk.

Confiscate Keys

If you're sober enough to realize that one of your friends is about to make a very bad decision, you should take responsibility and get in their way. That means taking their keys and offering to call them a cab or escort them to a public transportation station.

If you have been drinking at all, you should never offer to drive a friend home. You might be less drunk than them and more likely to safely operate a vehicle, but you could still be putting both your lives and the lives of others on the road at risk.

<u>Ways Your Community Can Prevent Drunk Driving</u>

Of course, it never hurts to have everyone rallying behind prevention plans. Legal ramifications are only so much of a deterrent when people convince themselves that they won't get caught. Communities, particularly those that have seen loss from drunk driving incidents, take a variety of measures to get the word out about drunk driving and to prevent further heartache.

Education

If you went to high school any time in the last twenty to thirty years, you've likely been subject to an assembly with human interest stories and heartbreaking monologues about drunk driving tragedy. Initiatives like these seek to deter drunk drivers not only by discussing legal ramifications, but also by humanizing statistics. Sometimes tugging at the heartstrings is the only way to get through to people who might otherwise not take a matter seriously.

Sobriety Checkpoints

A more practical preventative measure involves stopping all passing cars at various checkpoints along a road. Typically, sobriety checkpoints are located in areas where there may be high traffic late at night. Police may stop all or some vehicles to check for drunk drivers and administer breathalyzer and field sobriety tests whenever appropriate. This strategy may seem punitive, but it is effective. After all, if you are thinking of driving home drunk and you know there could be a sobriety checkpoint on your route, you don't have to wonder whether or not you'll get caught.

Ignition Interlocks

These devices prevent those who have been drinking from starting up their vehicles. They require drivers to pass a breathalyzer test. These devices can be court ordered for repeat drunk driving offenders. However, some people have argued for their universal use in any vehicle.

<u>Know Your Resources</u>

If you do find yourself in accident where either you or another driver was under the influence, then contact a lawyer and apprise yourself of your rights. Each state has its own set of laws on the books for how to handle these situations, and a good lawyer can help you navigate those muddy waters. You can also contact your local DMV or check out their website. Many have resources for both victims and perpetrators.

On November 6th 2012, Colorado passed Amendment 64 that effectively legalized marijuana within the state by outlawing its drug policy against the substance. This was largely considered a victory by those who thought marijuana laws were punitive, particularly against people of color or people of lower income demographics. However, it also presented some interesting new challenges.

Traffic fatalities have been on the rise in Colorado. In a report card recently released by the Colorado Department of Transportation (CDOT) , they noted a 12% increase in traffic deaths between 2014 and 2015. Since the releasing of the report, the department has received some flack. While the report mentions statistics on alcohol related crashes it notably doesn't mention marijuana.

Glenn Davis, manager of the CDOTs Highway Safety department acknowledges and admits that the technology exists to test drivers for marijuana, but law enforcement has been slow to adapt.

However, there is another reason why local authorities might be

finding it challenging to enforce laws against stoned driving.

Cole notes and others agree that the mere presence of marijuana in

someone's system is not proof that they were driving under the

influence. THC, the active ingredient in the drug, can linger in the

system for anywhere from five days to two months depending on

the amount and frequency of the marijuana consumption. Urine

and hair tests can detect the drug long after the individual is no

longer intoxicated. Even blood and saliva tests can sometimes test

positive for the drug days after consumption in heavier users.

This presents a complicated problem for law enforcement and not

only in Colorado. Alcohol is easy to focus on because it is

commonly used and easy to test for. Once it's out of your system,

it's gone. However, a multitude of drugs means a multitude of

tests and they may not all mean what we think they do. Add to this

the fact that many drivers under the influence of drugs may be suffering side effects or interactions from legal drug use, and

understanding and enforcing the muddy waters of drugged driving

is murky indeed.

<u>Drugged Driving Statistics</u>

Traffic Deaths

- As of 2010, roughly 4,000 drivers with drugs in their

  system die annually. This only includes drivers that were

  tested, meaning that the number could be much higher.

  (NHTSA)

- As of 2010, roughly 18% of driving related deaths involved

  people on drugs other than alcohol. (NHTSA)

Number of Drugged Drivers

- In 2013, nearly 10 million people admitted in a survey that they have driven while under the influence of drugs. (SAMHSA)

- A 2005 study determined that over half of drivers that were admitted to a Level-1 trauma center (for major injuries) had drugs in their system. (Accident Analysis and Preventation)

Drugged Driving Demographics

- Men are more likely to drive under the influence of drugs. (SAMHSA)

- Individuals between the ages of 18 and 24 are significantly more likely to drive under the influence of drugs. (SAMHSA)

- According to a 2010 study, drivers over the age of 50 accounted for more and a quarter of those in fatal crashes. (American Journal of Epidemiology)

Involving THC

- Drivers who tested positive for THC (the active ingredient in marijuana) increased about 47% between 2007 and 2014. This is a greater increase than with any other drug. (NHTSA Roadside Survey)

- Over one third of teenagers believe that marijuana makes them better drivers. (Liberty Mutual/SADD poll)

- Marijuana in combination with other drugs (like alcohol or cocaine) poses a greater risk than any of these drugs used alone, indicating that the interaction between marijuana and these drugs is of particular concern. (Public Health Report)

Involving Prescription Drugs

- According to a 2010 study, of drivers who have tested positive for drugs, 47% had used prescription drugs. (Public Health Report)

The Problem with Statistics

While the statistics noted above are certainly alarming, they should also be considered with a grain of salt. Drugged driving statistics are somewhat suspect, as they consider a wide range of substances with a wide variety of effects and interactions. For many of these drugs there are no reliable roadside tests that can confirm intoxication (note what we mentioned in the introduction about marijuana). What's more, police officers rarely test for additional drugs when they confirm the presence of alcohol in a driver's system, making it hard to know exactly how many drivers do so under the influence of drugs. Finally, when multiple drugs are confirmed, it's difficult to know which drugs played the largest role in impairment.

It's also worth mentioning that different demographics have statistically significant numbers of drugged drivers. The facts mentioned above tell us that those between the ages of 18 and 24 are more likely to drive under the influence of drugs. This might make sense if you consider that they are also more likely to experiment with recreational substances. However, the facts also tell us that those over the age of 50 play a larger role in drugged driving as well. It stands to reason that these drivers may have been experiencing side effects or interactions from prescription medications. Here we have two dramatically different groups lumped into the same category for drastically different reasons.

<u>Drugged Driving vs. Drunk Driving</u>

Why do we treat these separately? Isn't alcohol a drug after all? Historically, we've been more concerned with drunk driving because it seemed to be more prevalent. First of all, alcohol is a legal substance, making it more accessible to the general public. What's more, it's almost guaranteed to have a negative impact on one's ability to operate a vehicle, unlike many legal prescription or non-prescription medications. Finally, it's served in copious amounts at locations distant from one's home. Our societal norms have conjured a recipe for disaster.

Drugged driving has traditionally been less common. It's harder to get your hands on the kinds of drugs that would cause serious impairment. Additionally, many of these drugs are already illegal, so it seems superfluous to create and enforce a law that specifically addresses driving while under their influence. And once more, it's harder to test for their influence at the moment of driving, making it more difficult to hold up convictions in court.

However, the tides are turning. A report from the Governors Highway Safety Association (GHSA) concluded that drugs were associated with more driving deaths than alcohol in 2015. Of those motorists who died and were tested for substances, 43% had drugs in their system while only 37% had alcohol. Of course, this association is purely correlative and does not prove that those drivers were under the drug's influence at the time. However, it does raise some serious questions about the prevalence of drugged driving and makes many citizens wonder if we shouldn't be doing more to prevent it.

<u>Drugs Most Likely to Cause Accidents</u>

As with alcohol, any drug that is intended to alter your conscious state is a big no on the highway. We don't think we need to tell you that driving while on hallucinogens or similarly intense substances is going to get you nowhere good if you climb behind the wheel. However, you may not realize that even something as innocuous as over the counter pain killers can be a problem while driving. The following drugs have all been shown to have some effect on driving.

Sedatives

This one should be fairly straight-forward. The very nature of the problem is in the name. Sedatives cause drowsiness, dizziness, confusion, poor concentration, and delayed reactions. In other words, they sedate you.

Sedatives include over-the-counter sleep aids like Unisom and ZzzQuil. These drugs have diphenhydramine as an active ingredient. This antihistamine, like many others, causes drowsiness. They also include more intense prescription sleep aids.

Barbiturates are serious sedatives. These drugs enhance neurotransmitters that inhibit activity in the brain causing the sedative effect. Admittedly, they have largely been replaced by safer alternatives. But they may still be used in extreme cases, especially when treating seizures.

Benzodiazepines are essentially the new barbiturate. They are considered safer and harder to abuse, but they are still serious business and require a prescription. These tranquilizers include familiar names like Valium and Xanax. They typically aren't used as sleep aids so much as they are used to treat anxiety. This makes them particularly high risk for drivers as drivers may know better than to take sleep aids before driving but may not have the same consideration for their anti-anxiety meds.

Allergy and Cold Medication

We mentioned that the active ingredient in over-the-counter sleep aids is an antihistamine called diphenhydramine. Antihistamines do more than just makes you drowsy. They are used to treat allergic reactions. Drugs like Benadryl are used for seasonal allergies, rashes, and more. As such, these allergy meds have sedative qualities and could affect driving.

Cold medicine, on the other hand, may not make you drowsy unless it specifically has a sleep aid in it (like Nyquil). However, they can make you very loopy, which comes with its own host of problems. Depending on the cold medicine, too much can leave you distracted, jittery, and even cause a psychoactive reaction.

Painkillers

Don't worry, you're not likely to get into an accident if you pop some aspirin for a headache before you drive home from work. However, painkillers can often have unexpected effects on our bodies and it's important to know how yours affect you.

Let's start with the obvious. Prescription painkillers like Codeine, Vicodin, and the notorious Oxycontin are going to have a serious effect on your mental state. These drugs are all opioids, which cause severe drowsiness, slowed reaction time, and more.

However, a painkiller doesn't need to come with a prescription to affect your driving. At the right dosages, even Tylenol can cause you to lose concentration and feel sleepy. But don't worry, when we say "the right dose," we mean serious prescription-level doses.

Anti-Nausea and Antidepressants

This is our "other" category. It's simply worth noting that less commonly consumed drugs, like anti-nausea and antidepressants, can also have sedative qualities. It's always good to be cautious about the drugs you choose to take if you plan to get behind the wheel.

Stimulants

Finally, we want to look at drugs that don't cause drowsiness but may still affect driving. Stimulants include anything from caffeine to Ritalin. In many cases they are fine and can actually keep you awake. However, when taken in excess, stimulants can cause heart failure and seizures. The more intense the stimulant, the greater the risk.

How to Avoid Drugged Driving

With so many drugs and so many side effects, how can we be sure that we are driving safely? It's a good question. After all, you don't want to have to avoid the road for several hours or days every time you have a headache or cold. Thankfully, there are some precautionary measures you can take to stay safe.

- **Watch your dose.** This is not to say, "don't overdose." That much should be a given. This simply means that you shouldn't assume a drug that is fine at one dose will be fine at another. Let's say your doctor starts you on 20mg of an anti-anxiety medication. You feel fine on it. Great. Now he ups it to 30mg. It's time to slow down and make sure it's safe before you go driving.

- **Know how a drug affects you.** This is an extension of the last tip. Any time you are taking a new drug you need to give it time to work on you. Never go driving on a drug you haven't tested first.

- **Read about side effects.** Read the label. Look it up online. Just do what you have to do to make sure you understand the drug and all of its effects.

- **Know your interactions.** If you are planning on taking more than one drug (even if they're both over-the-counter medications) apprise yourself of any possible interactions.

Don't just assume that because they treat different conditions they have to do with different functions in the body and therefore have no relationship to one another. You'd be surprised.

- **Follow directions.** Does the medication say on the box "do not operate heavy machinery" or something to that affect? Then don't.

- **Try an evening dose.** If you take a medication daily that has a drowsy affect, then take it in the evenings when you're less likely to be driving. In many cases, doctors will advice patients to take these medications before bedtime.

- **Drugs don't make you a better driver.** This tip doesn't exactly fit with the others, but it's worth mentioning. Many people erroneously assume that because a drug makes them jittery or forces them to pay more attention that they are a more cautious and attentive driver. This is false. The best driver is one who is in total control.

<u>Medical Emergencies</u>

Sometimes certain medical conditions can affect driving regardless of the type of medication being taken. Anything from an asthma attack to a seizure will certainly take your mind of the road. To minimize the extent of an accident and any injuries involved, it's important to know the warning signs for any medical condition that you might reasonably expect to experience.

Seizure

Most people who experience seizures and are old enough to drive will be epileptic. Therefore, they should already know they are a risk factor. However, there are some rare instances where seizures can occur in non-epileptic people.

It's also worth noting that seizures tend to come on quickly and have varying degrees of warning. You won't have much time to respond, but if you're alert you may be able to just enough to avoid a serious accident.

Risk Factors

- Diagnosed epilepsy

- Diabetes (extremely low blood sugar)

- Very high fever

- Stroke (see below)

Warning signs

- Auditory aura (like music)

- Feeling of temperature change

- Blurry vision

- Muscle spasms

- Strange taste in mouth

- Clenching teeth

- Sense of losing consciousness

Stroke

While there are some risk factors for stroke, it is also possible for people without any risk factors and at a young age to experience a stroke due to congenital heart defects, blood clotting, and more. It is good to learn the warning signs for stroke regardless of how likely you are to have one.

Risk Factors

- High blood pressure

- Heart disease

- Obesity

- Diabetes

- Family history

- Age (the older you are the greater the risk)

- Gender (women are typically at a greater risk)

- Ethnicity (most common in people of African or Native American/Alaskan descent)

Warning signs

- Drooping or numbness in face

- Weakness or numbness in one arm

- Trouble speaking

- Trouble seeing in one or both eyes

- Sudden severe headache

Heart Attack

There is some overlap between heart attack and stroke and many people who are at a high risk for one are also at a high risk for the other.

Risk Factors

- Smoking

- High blood pressure

- High cholesterol

- Diabetes

- Family history

- Obesity

- Stress

- Some autoimmune conditions

Warning signs

- Pressure, tightness, or pain in the chest

- Pain that spreads to the back or shoulders

- Nausea

- Indigestion or heartburn

- Cold sweat

- Dizziness

Anaphylactic Shock

This extreme allergic reaction typically results from exposure to a food, insect venom, or medication allergen. The first step in avoiding accidents due to anaphylactic shock is to avoid the allergens that cause it. However, that's not always possible.

Risk Factors

- Food allergies (nuts, fish, shellfish, etc.)

- Insect allergies (bee stings, fire ants, etc.)

- Medication allergies (antibiotics, painkillers, etc.)

- Some topical allergens (latex, certain plants, etc.)

Warning signs

- Flushing

- Hives

- Swelling in throat or mouth

- Difficulty speaking

- Asthma like symptoms

- Nausea or vomiting

- Changes in heart rate

- Sense of impending doom

If you think you are experiencing any of these conditions, it's important that you slow your vehicle and attempt to pull off the road. You should also try to put your hazards on as an indication to other drivers that they should watch out for your vehicle. Do not speed up for any reason, even if your close to a rest stop or home. If there must be an accident, one at slower speeds will result in fewer injuries.

<u>Legal Ramifications</u>

Put simply, you are responsible when there is a reasonable expectation that you could have avoided the situation. In other words, if you knew that a medication would likely affect you a certain way and chose to drive anyway, then you are responsible for any accidents that occur as a result of your altered state.

The same is true if you are aware of any drug interactions or are disobeying your doctor's orders in regard to a medical condition. Finally, different states may have different laws on the books for when you are allowed to drive under certain conditions (like having to be seizure free for a set period of time). All the more reason to educate yourself about any drugs you're taking or

conditions you might have. Keep yourself and others safe.

Chapter Four: Fatigued Driving

You probably remember the tragic accident that killed comedian James McNair and nearly took the life of Tracy Morgan. The popular SNL and 30 Rock actor narrowly survived and spent several years recovering from the psychological and physical trauma caused by the crash.

You may not remember Kevin Roper, the Walmart truck driver who hit Morgan's limousine on the New Jersey Turnpike. Roper was eventually charged with first-degree aggravated manslaughter, second-degree vehicular homicide, and third-degree aggravated assault charges, all of which he plead guilty to. His crime? He was too tired to be on the road, let alone behind the wheel of a commercial truck.

Of course, Roper had been up for a reported 28 hours. According to court testimony, he'd actually driven 12 whole hours just to get to his 14-hour shift. Obviously, the average person is not going to be driving under these same conditions. However, fatigued driving is a real thing. Nurses coming down off of late night 12 hour shifts have to drive home. Parents who have been up all night with a fussy newborn have to make it to the grocery store. Sometimes, we're just too worn out to drive, but we do it anyway.

Now we know there are real consequences too. If a court determines that you should have known better, that you were acting recklessly or irresponsibly when you chose to drive, you could and likely will be held accountable for your actions. And saying you were too tired to know better won't get you very far. Just try that excuse in DUI court and see how far it gets you.

<u>Fatigued Driving Stats</u>

Fatigued Driving and Accidents

- Fatigued driving is the main cause of some 100,000 reported vehicle crashes every year. (NHTSA)

- Fatigued driving plays a role in about 328,000 crashes annually. (AAA)

- There were 83,000 crashes related to drowsy driving between 2005 and 2009. (NHTSA)

Fatigued Driving and Deaths/Injuries

- Fatigued driving kills at least 1,500 people a year and injures 71,000 more. (NHTSA)

- Fatigued driving makes up about 17% of crashes annually in which a person was hospitalized. (AAA)

- There were 846 deaths related to fatigued driving in 2014. (NHTSA)

Number of Fatigued Drivers

- 4.2% of people reported being drowsy while driving within the past 30 days. (CDC)

- 37% of people reported nodding off or falling asleep while behind the wheel. (2002 Gallup Poll)

- 7.5 million drivers nodded off in a given month. (2002 Gallup Poll)

- About 5% of adults admit to sleeping behind the wheel. (Accident Analysis and Prevention)

Fatigued Driving and Teens

- Teens who regularly sleep less than 8 hours a night at 1/3 more likely to get into an accident. (NHTSA)

- Teens need more than 9 hours of sleep a night to appropriately reduce the risk of fatigued driving. (National Sleep Foundation)

- Drivers under the age of 25 cause the majority of crashes in which fatigue was a factor. (National Sleep Foundation)

<u>How Does Fatigue Affect Your Driving</u>

Randy Gardner holds the record for the longest a human being has intentionally gone without sleep. Randy received this honor when he was a teenager in 1965. He elected to go without sleep to find out exactly what happened to the body and mind when they became dramatically sleep-deprived. His experiment lasted for precisely 264.4 hours, or 11 days and 24 minutes and it revealed some startling effects. After only a couple of days, Randy's eyes stopped focusing and he lost the ability to identify familiar objects from touch. Shortly after that, he became extremely moody and uncoordinated. After several more days, he could barely concentrate and had difficulty forming short-term memories. By the end of the experiment, he was paranoid and hallucinating. Sleep deprivation had driven him to psychosis. Thankfully, he was able to get his much needed rest and suffered no long term ill effects from the experiment, but many scientists count him lucky and don't recommend that any individual seek to break his record.

Obviously, your average sleep deprived person won't have stayed up for nearly as long as Randy did. In fact, they may be getting some sleep every night, just not enough. Therefore, there's little worry that they'll be careening down the road at fifty miles per hour while hallucinating, although it's not impossible. Why then are we sharing this with you? Randy's experiment is a testament to how much our bodies rely on sleep. It's not a matter of feeling better or more wakeful. It is, in some cases literally, a matter of life and death.

Our Brain Needs Sleep

When you sleep, it may seem like your brain is resting, but it's actually hard at work. Sleeping helps us turn short term memory into long term memory, as well as consolidate older memories. It's basically time for the brain to get organized before the next big day. A 2007 study from the University of California at Berkeley also suggested that sleep is a time for the brain to get creative. It would seem that in its nightly organization ritual, the brain is able to make connections between seemingly unconnected ideas, suggesting that sleep is pivotal when it comes to problem solving and "thinking outside of the box."

While scientists have long known the benefits of sleep for memory, problem solving, and concentration, they've recently discovered a much more specific function that may clue us in to the true purpose of sleep. In 2012, researchers at the University of Rochester Medical Center discovered something they termed the glymphatic system. This discovery not only answered some key questions about our need for rest, but also addressed another mystery involving the brain.

"Waste clearance is of central importance to every organ," says Dr. Maiken Nedergaard of Rochester University's Center for Translational Neuromedicine, "and there have been long-standing questions about how the brain gets rid of its waste." The glymphatic system does exactly that. During the day, our brains accumulate waste. Much of this waste comes in the form of Adenosine, the chemical that makes us feel sleepy. This is also the chemical whose receptors are blocked by caffeine, making us wakeful. When we sleep, the glymphatic system releases cerebral spinal fluid into the brain, washing away the waste like a power washer rinsing dirt off a porch. If we don't get enough sleep, this waste can build up over time. With waste built up between brain cells, preventing them from functioning to their fullest potential, we can experience memory problems, concentration problems, problems with regulating our emotions, and even hallucinations. Remember Randy Gardner? He had a brain full of waste, and it was literally making him crazy.

As we've already mentioned, it's unlikely that your average sleep deprived individual would experience symptoms as extreme as Randy's. However, there are still consequences to getting too little sleep. Sleep deprivation affects our ability to learn new things, our ability to remember basic things, our mood, our ability to reason, and our reaction time. It's little wonder that poor sleep leads to poor driving.

Our Bodies Need Sleep

While the brain itself is most affected by sleep deprivation, it is not the only part of the body that relies on those precious nighttime hours. During sleep, our DNA works hard at repairing itself, helping us heal if we're injured. Our muscles relax and our body rests, boosting our immune system and helping us feel better if we're sick. Lack of sleep puts stress on the muscles and body, causing high blood pressure, muscle inflammation, and more. Sleep has also been linked to blood sugar levels and metabolism, lack of sleep putting us at greater risk of diabetes and obesity.

Probably the most concerned statistic when it comes to lack of sleep and your body is that sleep deprivation can put you at a dramatically increased risk of a stroke. People who regularly get fewer than six hours of sleep a night are 4 times more likely to have a stroke. Those already at risk of stroke might find that sleep deprivation is enough to push them over the edge. This is what happened to a soccer fan in 2014 who stayed up for roughly 48 hours to watch the World Cup. He died of a stroke as a result of his enthusiasm for the sport.

What Happens When We Drive

This is all well and good, but is a little sleep deprivation really going to be that bad for your driving? After all, you've driven to work after late nights and had no problems. You didn't nod off at the wheel even once. The truth is fatigued driving isn't just about falling asleep at the wheel, although that is a significant concern; it's about more subtle deficiencies that result from the lack of sleep. Remember that your brain was not able to properly rid itself of waste and now there's stuff getting in the way of those neurons firing. So if you've pounded the caffeine and don't feel drowsy in the slightest, that doesn't mean that your four hours of sleep last night aren't impacting you.

Fatigued drivers might feel fine, but they are likely experiencing any of the following:

- Impaired coordination

- Slow reaction time

- Impaired judgement

- Impaired memory

- Inability to effectively process information

- Difficulty focusing the eyes (and the brain)

- Mind wandering

- Irritability and impatience

Picture yourself driving at a decent clip down a familiar road. You know the turns so well that you take them almost on auto-pilot. The light ahead of your turns yellow, but you're too busy thinking about your sister's baby shower and how anxious you are about your gift. You definitely saw the light, but your brain didn't have the juice to register it and bring you back to the present. When you finally realize you're about to run a red, you slam the breaks a tad too late and run into a car on the cross-street. This is fatigued driving in its mildest form. In more extreme cases, you might be so tired that the lines on the road blur and you start to drift. You might be so tired that you nod of completely and awake with your car wrapped around a tree.

Fatigued Driving vs. Drunk Driving

Hmmm. Blurred vision. Impaired judgement. Poor memory. Poor reaction time. Even irritability. Does any of this sound familiar? Researchers have actually studied the similarities between fatigue driving and drunk driving. Studies show that being awake for even just 18 hours (6am to midnight) can make you drive like someone with a blood alcohol level of .05. If you recall from our chapter on drunk driving, that's about the point where your vision starts to weave and you're feeling brave enough to hit on the bartender. It may not be illegal yet as drunk driving goes, but it's not a good place to be when you're in charge of a giant machine.

How Driving Makes You Tired

Sometimes we feel fine when we get behind the wheel. We're well rested and rearing to go. But we have a long drive ahead of us and the driving itself starts to wear us down. Of course, anyone would get tired if they've been driving for 12 straight hours. But did you know that driving can actually make you tired more quickly? It seems strange, because we're not really moving our bodies much when we drive, but the act has an exhausting effect on our brains.

- **Repetition** – Driving is repetitive in a lot of ways. We stop. We go. We stop. We go. If we are driving a familiar route, like our route home from work, we go through all of the same motions that we do every single day. While this kind of repetition doesn't ask much of our brains or bodies, it doesn't stimulate our brain either.

- **Boredom** – This goes hand in hand with repetition. When our brains aren't stimulated, they can try to stimulate themselves, making our minds wander or making us stress out about unimportant things. This restlessness can be exhausting.

- **Lack of movement** – I know, it seems hard to believe that not moving much would possibly make you more tired than moving a little bit. But if you've ever worked an office job that had you behind a desk for eight or more hours a day, then you know all about this. Right around two in the afternoon, you're angling for the coffee maker because you're already yawing and nodding off at your computer.

- **Lack of food** – This one is a little more straight-forward. Food is fuel. Like stimulation and movement, too much can make us tired, but too little will also wear us down. If you've been driving for a while, you probably haven't eaten recently.

Highway Hypnosis

You teach at a high school some thirty minutes away from your house. You're up every morning at around 5am, so you can get to the school by 7am. You've driven this same route for years; you could probably handle it with your eyes closed. It's early and you're groggy, but you somehow manage to get showered and into the car. The next thing you remember, you're pulling onto the street that runs in front of the school. Where did the time go? Did you actually come all this way? Why don't you remember? You can't even recall what was playing on the radio.

This phenomenon is called highway hypnosis or white line fever. It's most common in truckers, but it can happen to anyone who drives regularly, especially on a familiar route. It's when your brain essentially runs on autopilot, taking you through the motions without your being conscious of anything. Your eyes see the lights, stop signs, and turns. Your brain responds appropriately, breaking, accelerating, and signaling. However, the part of you that's "present," well, isn't.

This is far more likely to happen when you're fatigued. Morning commutes and long road trips are the most likely culprits. It's a trance-like state, much like sleeping itself, and was famously referred to as "sleeping with the eyes open" in a 1929 study of the phenomenon. If you were to look at someone under its spell, they would likely be staring at a fixed point on the road with little expression on their face.

What's the big deal? I mean, if you're able to obey the traffic laws, then does it really matter if you "zone" for a while? Sure, you can handle a red light or a car breaking gradually in front of you, but highway hypnosis is ill-equipped to deal with more abrupt driving events that require greater presence of mind and faster reaction time. If someone brakes hard in front of you or runs a stop sign, you're probably going to get into an accident. Additionally, you might find yourself inadvertently driving much higher than the speed-limit or tailgating, further increasing your chances of an accident.

Stay Awake While Driving

You'll notice that many of the tips for preventing fatigue and combating existing fatigue are the same. Basically, you should use anti-fatigue strategies well before they become truly necessary. After all, a caffeine boost is only going to be so helpful when you're already nodding off at the wheel. Planning ahead will make you better able to withstand longer and later trips.

Tips for Preventing Fatigue and Highway Hypnosis

- **Get enough sleep.** It stands to reason that the less sleep you get, the more likely you are to doze off at inappropriate times. Get between 7 and 8 hours of sleep at night for safer driving during the day.

- **Avoid driving in the very early hours of the morning.**
  According to the National Sleep Foundation, people should
  avoid driving between midnight and 6am to avoid fighting
  their natural rhythms. Of course, this is not always
  avoidable.

- **Use rest stops.** They are called rest stops for a reason. We
  do actually need to rest from driving, especially on long
  trips.

- **Listen to talk radio.** You can try listening to music,
  especially if you're doing something active like singing
  along. But know that some music can contribute to the
  hypnotic effect of the road. Talk radio will stimulate you
  without any of the rhythmic repetition.

- **Take a food and water break.** When you are at that rest
  stop, eat something and get hydrated. Give your body more
  fuel to burn.

- **Drive with a friend.** Carpool to work. Bring a friend or two along for your road trip. Having people to talk to will help keep you stimulated. Just make sure they don't distract you. What's more, if you get too tired, someone else can take over.

- **Drink caffeine.** That caffeine buzz could mean the difference between nodding off into an accident and getting to your destination safely. If you know you're in for a long trip, get some coffee.

Tips for Staying Awake When You Feel Tired

- **Stop and rest.** This goes hand in hand with using rest stops. Except, instead of using them to preempt exhaustion, it's now time to admit that you're done driving for a while and you need a break. If it's late enough and you've been driving for several hours, you may even need a nap. We cover naps in more detail below.

- **Get engaged.** If you weren't already listening to talk radio or chatting with your carpool friend, now's the time to begin. True, engaging conversations might distract from driving, but when you're really tired, they could be enough to keep your brain awake. And let's face it, that's more important.

- **Play a game.** This extension of "get engaged" deserves its own mention. Road games are great for passing the time, but they can be even better for staying awake. Obviously, you don't want to play anything that's going to distract you too much from the road. But a simple word game or memory game while driving could help boost alertness.

- **Eat and Drink.** Enough said. If you drink something, make it cold with caffeine. You could also try a mint to stimulate your senses.

Recognize the Signs of Exhaustion

If you experience any of the following while driving, take immediate measures to wake yourself up or get off the road.

- Blinking a lot

- Eyes feel strained or heavy

- Closing your eyes more

- Yawning

- Driving errors

- Restlessness

- Irritability

- Wandering thoughts

<u>Sleeping on the Road</u>

You're on a long trip and you've been trying to stay awake long enough to make it to the next motel. However, that Cloud 9 you have your eye on is still over 20 miles away and you have reached your limit. It may be tempting to try and push yourself to make it the whole way, but you'd be putting yourself at undo risk.

Sometimes, you just have to phone it in and find someplace to pull over for a few hours of shut eye.

Can you really do that? Just pull over to the side of the road, turn off your car, kick back your seat, and snooze? Won't some cop come snooping around, thinking you're up to no good? Worse yet, will you get robbed or axe murdered?

First of all, this is not as strange a concept as it might sound. Believe it not, cars were at one point specifically designed with the expectation that people would be sleeping in them. Cars designed in the 1940's, 50's, and 60's all had seats that thoroughly reclined, allowing for maximum car sleeping comfort. Advertisements even showed young families sharing a sleeping space in the back of their car, making a Kodak moment out of what some people might consider a harrowing prospect.

Of course, times have changed. Sleeping in cars is not nearly as mainstream as it once was. It has gone by the wayside much like hitchhiking and similarly questionable traditions. Conflicting laws and heightened fear over "drifters" have deterred people from these practices. That being said, it is still possible, and sometimes necessary, to sleep in your car.

Is it Legal to Sleep in Your Car?

Let's begin with the question of legality. Whether or not it's legally OK to pull over and sleep in your car depends on the city or state in question. It also sometimes depends on the circumstances and your condition.

In many states, it's legal to sleep in your car as long as you are not obstructing traffic. However, many cities restrict sleeping in cars at certain times of the day or at all. Often these laws are intended to deter the homeless population from sticking around, but they will apply to you as well. If you're outside of city limits, you're subject to state or county laws.

In some states or counties, it's OK to sleep in your car as long as you are at a rest stop and / or not under the influence of drugs or alcohol. You'll recall from out section on drunk driving that you can be convicted of drunk driving if you are drunk and inside of a vehicle whether or not it's actually moving.

Given these murky legal waters, it may just make more sense to avoid citation altogether and pull into a rest stop or campground. This will get you safely off the road and give you a private space with which to take your nap or spend the night. If you're planning a road trip, apprise yourself of the campgrounds and rest stops along the way. Even if you're not banking on spending the night in your Subaru, it can't hurt to know your options.

Is it Safe to Sleep in Your Car?

This question is a little trickier. Laws provide hard and fast guidelines for what is or is not going to get you into trouble. However, cops aren't the only ones you're going worry about when pulling into a secluded spot in the middle of the night.

Many people may feel reticent about pulling into an empty campsite at one in the morning for fear that they'll be the subject of violent crime. The truth is, scenarios involving homicidal drifters and couples huddled in their Buick in the dark are fueled by crime dramas and horror movies. In reality, random murders or robberies in rural spots are rare at best.

If you're concerned about having a gun pulled on you when you're trying to get some shut eye, avoid urban areas, especially those with high crime. You're far more likely to be the object of violence in these high-crime and high-population areas than you are at a rest stop thirty miles outside of the city.

What you don't want to do is work yourself up into a frenzy. That will keep you from getting those precious Z's, and isn't why you're doing this in the first place?

How to Sleep Comfortably

If you are heading out on a long trip and know there's a chance you'll be pulling into a motel for some sleep, prepare for the possibility that you might be sleeping in your car instead. That means bringing overnight supplies for the experience.

- **Bedding** – You don't need to go overboard here, but do plan to bundle up. Some areas of the country can get cold at night and you won't be running the heat in your car unless you want to wake up to a dead battery.

- **Sleeping Pad** – Technically, this could qualify as bedding, but it's worth its own mention. Believe it or not, cars are not all that comfortable to sleep in (especially modern designs).

- **Provisions** – If you're planning to be stopped for a while, you'll likely get hungry or tired. In particular, make sure you have water available.

- **First Aid Kit** – This might sound a bit extreme. However, if you're planning a long trip, then it can't hurt to have one on hand for those long stretches of road between towns. The same can be said for any night spent in seclusion.

- **Fully Charged Electronics** – If you're on the road for a long period of time, you'll want to bring a phone charger as it is. Make sure your phone is juiced for your overnight stint in the car. It is essential in case of an emergency but will also be helpful if you need to set an alarm.

Of course, having supplies is only part of the puzzle. You also need to find a way to actually sleep in the car. If your car has a back seat that can be layed forward, then your best bet is to flatten the back as much as possible and stretch out with your blankets. That may require some rearranging if you've got a lot of luggage with you, but it'll be worth it for a better night's sleep. You can always sleep in the front if you have to, but be prepared for a stiff neck and a particularly restless night.

Use Your Best Judgement

Do we recommend that you plan to sleep in your car? Not really. Some people swear by it, and it will certainly save you money, but there are risks involved and the quality of your sleep will likely be poor. However, a citation and a stiff neck are superior to running yourself off the road because you were too exhausted to keep your eyes open. Weigh your options, and get off the road if you don't feel safe driving.

How Much Sleep Do You Really Need?

We've spent a lot of time talking about the importance of getting enough sleep, but we haven't really talked about what that actually means. After all, "enough sleep" for a ten-year-old is not the same as it is for someone in their thirties. As we get older, our bodies need less sleep to thrive. However, many adults still don't get nearly enough.

According to the Center for Disease Control (CDC), about a third of all American adults don't get enough sleep. The National Sleep Foundation reports that 45% of American adults feel that poor sleep affects their daily lives. The problem isn't just endemic to America. A 2016 poll concluded that the average UK adult was sleeping an hour shy of what they need. This corroborated a 2016 study by Benson for Beds that concluded the average UK adult was missing out on an entire night of sleep each week. In fact, the United Kingdom is listed as the most sleep deprived country according to a study by Aviva, an international insurance company. It's followed by Ireland, Canada, and the United States.

How much sleep is enough? The National Sleep Foundation lists the following breakdown for sleep ranges by age. Understanding that every individual is different, the National Sleep Foundation provides wide ranges for what may be acceptable. However, the typical range is highly recommended for individuals.

- Newborn (0-3 months)
  - Wide range: 11-19
  - Typical range: 14-17
- Infant (4-11 months)
  - Wide range: 10-18
  - Typical range: 12-15
- Toddler (1-2 years)
  - Wide range: 9-16
  - Typical range: 11-14
- Preschool (3-5 years)
  - Wide range: 8-14
  - Typical range: 10-13
- School Age (6-13 years)
  - Wide range: 7-12
  - Typical range: 9-11

- Teenager (14-17 years)

    o Wide range: 7-11

    o Typical range: 8-10

- Young Adult (18-25 years)

    o Wide range: 6-11

    o Typical range: 7-9

- Adult (26-64 years)

    o Wide range: 6-10

    o Typical range: 7-9

- Older Adult (Over 65 years)

    o Wide range: 5-9

    o Typical range: 7-8

Make-Up Sleep Won't Help You

We know what you're thinking. It doesn't matter if you average

six hours a night during the week as long as you make up for it on

the weekend. This mentality is popular among college students and young professionals who pride themselves in their ability to push the limits and then sleep until noon on Saturday. The truth is that make-up sleep is not as effective as you might hope. Sure, it's better than nothing. Obviously, your body is craving sleep and you're giving it what it needs. In that sense, getting make-up sleep is better than continuing to average six hours a night. However, it's not better than just getting the right amount of sleep on a regular basis.

A 2013 study published in the American Journal of Physiology studied the restorative effects of make-up sleep. The researchers measured the physical and mental effects of poor sleep and make-up sleep in a range of individuals. They determined that cortisol, the stress hormone, had gone down, suggesting that the make-up sleep did have some immediate restorative effects on the body. However, the mental effects of poor sleep were little changed. The research suggested that individuals would need longer sleep more regularly to fully restore them.

Take heed, especially in you drive for a living. You may feel better after an 11-hour power sleep, but your crazy sleep schedule is still wreaking long term havoc on your system, making you generally less focused, less energized, and less in control.

Chapter Five: Distracted Driving

I sometimes reminisce fondly about days gone by when I left for work in the morning and was out of communication until I returned home in the late afternoon. How did we ever survive? Of course there are numerous benefits to this age of instant communications, including the benefit of being able to summon assistance when necessary during a drive. But think about it and be honest. How many times when you make and take those calls while driving did you really have to make and take those calls, or could the calls have waited until you reached your destination? I think you see the point.

Remember Carlee Bollig, who killed Charles Maurer and his daughter when she ran a red because she was distracted by her cell phone. Her case was open and shut, and she plead guilty to criminal vehicular homicide. Cell phones are the classic example of distracted driving and with good reason. According to the National Safety Council, cell phone use while driving causes about 1.6 million crashes a year. With the advent of the smartphone and the prevalence of texting, more and more people are finding it hard to keep their eyes off their screens and on the road.

Of course, cell phones aren't the only culprit. Technology in general as proven troublesome on the road, and much of it is more egregious than you might think. In 2016, a London biker caught a woman on film who had her laptop propped up in her passenger seat and was typing while stopped at a red light. True, the woman was stopped at a red light, a fact that she repeatedly pointed out to the biker, but one has to wonder why she was so incapable of putting the computer aside and whether her incessant need to interact with it could cause her to glance its way while the car was in motion.

This scene raises a much larger question. Why are we so obsessed with our technology? How have our lives gotten to the point where we can't make a simple commute home without staying completely connected? Part of it is likely a desensitization to the affect that these tools have on us.

We'll also pay homage to non-technological forms of distracted driving. After all, technology use is not the only form of distracted driving that we're faced with. Distractions can be simple and seemingly innocuous. They can also be largely out of our control.

In this chapter, we'll explore all kinds of distracted driving. We'll also examine our tumultuous relationship with technology and the internet and how they may contribute to distracted driving.

<u>Distracted Driving Stats</u>

Note that the following statistics are somewhat suspect given inconsistency with the use of the term "distracted driving." Distracted driving could involve friends or children causing disruptions or physically interacting with the driver. It could also involve distractions on the road like bright lights or roadside displays. The sources for the following stats don't always specify what they mean by "distracted driving" and often use the term "distracted driving" when only referring to technology, cell phones, or even just texting. As a result, the actual numbers for all types of distracted driving could be significantly higher than those listed here.

Accidents Caused

- Driving while texting leads to about 1.6 million crashes a year. (National Safety Council)

- Roughly 330,000 injuries occur a year from texting while driving.

- A quarter of all car accidents that happen in the United States involve texting while driving.

- Texting is 6 times more likely to result in a car accident than alcohol.

- Teens are more likely than adults to get into accidents while using a cell phone (texting or talking) by a factor of four.

- 3,154 people were killed from distracted driving related crashed in 2013.

A Survey of Drivers

- 94% of drivers want to ban texting while driving.

- 74% of drivers want to ban holding a cell phone at all when driving.

- 94% of teens recognize that texting while driving is bad. (AAA)

- 35% of those teens who recognize it as bad will do it anyway. (AAA)

<u>Types of Distracted Driving</u>

Before we go any further, let's be clear about what we mean when we talk about distracted driving. This is a broad category that includes, technology, friends and even billboard signs. In short, distracted driving is when your driving is impeded not by altered mental states (as from substances, lack of sleep, etc.), but from your external environment.

- **Texting** – This should go without saying at this point. Texting while driving has become the poster child for distracted driving and the type most people are keen to talk about.

- **Other Cell Phone Use** – Although texting seems to be the largest concern, it's not the only thing people use their phones for on the road. Internet use, social media use, and even just talking on the phone with eyes on the road lead to distraction.

- **Tablets and Laptops** – Tablet and laptop use are far less common than phone use. Let's face it, smartphones are basically tiny computers as it is and far less unwieldy in a vehicle. However, as the anecdote at the start of this chapter indicates, some people will still go all out with their technology use behind the wheel.

- **Radio Displays** – You might be surprised to see this listed here. After all, radio displays come with the car. Would they really give you something that wasn't safe to use? Understand that anything that takes your eyes of the road even for a few seconds or a hand off the wheel is distracting you from the task of driving. Shuffling through stations and pushing buttons counts as distracted driving.

- **GPS Navigation** – Here's another one you might be a little surprised to see. Isn't GPS specifically designed to be used while driving? Isn't that the whole point? Once again, looking at your GPS navigation display will take your eyes off the road. Sure, most people with GPS displays will offer it a quick glance to see how far away their next turn is, and truth be told, it's hardly as distracting as texting and won't necessarily require you to take your hands off the wheel. However, it is still a distraction and too much fussing with it could cause an accident. Be cognizant of that fact when using GPS and, if you have a passenger, allow them to read the directions to you.

- **Carpool** – This really depends on who you're carpooling with. If your passengers are well-behaved, then there really shouldn't be a problem. However, if your passengers are rowdy and not behaving in a safe manner, there could be a big problem. Engaging in conversation is OK as long as you don't let yourself get worked up and forget the most important thing you're doing.

- **Backseat (or Side-seat) Drivers** – Yes, yes, we did say to have a passenger manage the navigation system if you can. But that's not really what we mean by a backseat driver. A backseat driver is definitively someone who provides unsolicited, and often unhelpful, directions or insists on arguing with you about directions or your driving. They'll shout at you to slow down when they see a red in the distance. They'll say things like "turn now, turn now" when you're trying to make a left. They'll lecture you on how fast or slow you're going. In short, they are annoying and their sometimes aggressive directions can be alarming, stressful, and , you guessed it, distracting.

- **Young Children** – Here is a distraction that often can't be helped. If you have an infant who is incessantly screaming in their seat, you just have to train yourself to stay focused on your driving until you can find a safe place to pull off the road and tend to their needs. As they get older, kids could start throwing things, kicking the back of your seat, or messing with the power windows. Later, we'll go into more depth on how to manage misbehaving children in the car.

- **Eating and Drinking** – Ok, so this one isn't necessarily as bad as the others. Besides, eating or drinking something is one way to help keep yourself awake and energized on the road. However, it's important to understand how busy hands are not hands on the wheel and certain types of messy or hot foods can be hazardous when consumed in a car.

- **Roadside Distractions** – Not all distractions are inside of your vehicle. Everything from roadside accidents to flashy billboards can draw your eyes away from the road. It's important to stay focused on the task at hand.

<u>Our Relationship with Technology and the Slippery Slope</u>

When the internet was still finding its voice in the 90s and early 2000s, people spoke at length about internet addiction. It mattered that individuals were spending a few hours a day staring at a backlit screen, surfing the web or exploring chat rooms. These days, a few hours on the internet feel like nothing at all. Between work, social media, games, and other tools, people are spending anywhere from a few hours to most of their waking day on the net. However, internet and technology addiction is still a real thing and could be a major contributor to technology use at inappropriate times, like when operating a vehicle.

The Power of Internet Addiction

In the spring of 2017, NPR highlighted the story of one woman and her internet addicted daughter. The daughter, once sociable and outgoing, had become withdrawn, spending hours at night just staring at her phone. Many people, parents included, might be tempted to write this off as typical teen behavior. After all, isn't the teenaged girl with the cell phone permanently attached to her hand a popular stereotype? However, just because the culprit is a piece of tech doesn't mean it isn't causing significant mood changes and a drop in academic performance. In fact, psychiatrists have likened this type of behavior to that of drug or alcohol addicted individuals.

Kimberly Young wrote in a 2010 article in World Psychiatry about her own discoveries regarding internet addiction. She mentioned being inspired to write her 1998 book, *Caught in the Net*, when a friend announced that she would be divorcing her husband over his incessant chat room use. *Caught in the Net* went on to be the first book to really broach the subject of internet addiction, lending a voice to the suffering that many had already become intimately familiar with.

In her article, she cites a 2006 study published in CNS Spectrums, which concludes that one in every eight Americans show signs of "problematic internet use." With this firmly in mind, she calls for a greater understanding of the scope of the problem, suggesting that internet addiction continues to be an undervalued and poorly identified social problem.

Recognizing Internet Addiction

Can there really be so many internet addicted adults out there?

Note that the aforementioned study talks about adults that "show signs" of internet addiction. Like most things, internet dependence and addiction is on a spectrum. Showing one or two signs of addiction is not necessarily indicative of a serious problem. However, it should give you pause and suggests that you or your loved one may need to consider making some changes before a minor issue becomes a major one.

Physical Signs of Internet Addiction:

- **Backache** - This would be from sitting at a computer for too long. It may also result from poor posture while hunching over a cellular phone.

- **Headache** – This is a common problem from looking too long or too closely at backlit screens.

- **Changes in weight** – Weight gain could result from too much time spent being sedentary or the tendency to snack while browsing the internet. Internet browsing could also mean weight loss if the individual is so distracted by their phone or computer that they neglect to eat.

- **Changes in sleep patterns** – Many internet addicted individuals have a tendency to browse the web late into the evening, causing them to stay up later than they might otherwise. Backlit screens also have a waking effect, making it easier for them to stay awake at odd hours.

- **Changes in vision** – Screens are bad for the eyes. There's no arguing this point. Optometrists frequently recommend that individuals take brakes during work, allowing their eyes to rest by focusing on something in the distance. Too much screen time can cause eyesight to deteriorate.

- **Carpal Tunnel Syndrome** – This is a risk for anyone who spends a lot of time on a computer typing and clicking with a mouse. It doesn't have to be exclusive to those with an internet use addiction.

Behavioral Signs of Internet Addiction:

- **Isolation** – Internet addicted people will withdraw. They will be more focused on the virtual world than they are on loves ones. They may even physically isolate themselves if they feel the outside world is interfering with their internet use.

- **Lying** – Under "Emotional Signs of Internet Addiction," you'll notice the word "guilt." Lying stems from this. Many internet addicted individuals secretly or subconsciously understand that the amount of time they are spending on the internet is inappropriate and lie to loved ones in order to cover it up. This could mean lying about the amount of time they spend on the internet or lying about the types of activities they engage in. For example, someone who spent the last few hours on YouTube might lie and say they spent that time working.

- **Unreliability** – Internet addicted people have poor time management. Often hours can feel like minutes when they are "stuck" online. As a result, they tend to miss scheduled appointments and forget to do things that they've promised to do.

- **Developing emotional connections with people online** – There is nothing inherently wrong with making a connection online. Many people look for companionship, understanding, and commiseration on social media, forums, and more. Just because your loved one has made an online connection doesn't mean they have a problem. However, internet addicted individuals are more prone to this sort of connection and will often spend more time talking with or about their online friend than their physical friends.

- **Problems in your relationship** – Spending more time online means spending less time with loved ones. Internet addicted individuals will often find their physical relationships deteriorate even as their online ones thrive. For those who care about an internet addicted person, it may seem like the only way to communicate with them is through technology.

Emotional Signs of Internet Addiction:

- **Guilt** – Note what we said about lying. Those with an internet addiction often sense it. They may feel guilty about their behavior and seek to hide it. They may also try to rationalize their behavior to themselves, constantly working to convince themselves that they spend a normal amount of time on their computer or phone.

- **Defensiveness** – Although internet addicted people may secretly recognize the problem with their behavior, they will likely remain unwilling to admit it to others. When confronted, they will lie and behave defensively.

- **Anxiety** – This goes hand in hand with guilt. When they know secretly that they have a problem, they may experience anxiety or tension at the thought of being "found out." Anxiety can also occur when internet addicted people are forced to unplug, whether because they internet is down, they are traveling, or something else.

- **Depression** – Along with anxiety comes depression. Internet addiction breeds shame and a decreased sense of self-worth. Often these feelings exacerbate the issue by causing the individual to escape into the internet rather than face their own feelings.

- **Comfort or euphoria when online** – If depression and anxiety cause internet addicted people to escape into the internet, then it's because the internet offers some relief.

- **Loss of control** – One of the most reliable signs of addiction is the inability to manage one's own actions. If you repeatedly resolve to spend less time on the internet and find that you repeatedly fail to keep that resolution, then you might be an internet addict.

Internet Addiction and Distracted Driving

While all of the signs and symptoms mentioned above are essential for understanding internet addiction, let's take some time to focus on anxiety. Have you ever felt naked without your cell phone in hand? Have you ever found yourself without service and noticed the boredom and restlessness setting in? If so, you're not necessarily addicted to the internet, but you might have some idea what it feels like for internet addicts to be prevented from going online.

They might experience a profound boredom or sense of dread. More likely, they'll feel frustrated, depressed, and anxious. They'll have a compulsive need to go online and do, well, anything. Now picture that addict driving. Someone who can't make a fifteen-minute trip without texting friends, looking up song lyrics, or just reading the news is quite possibly an addict.

Don't get us wrong. We are not trying to absolve anyone of responsibility for their actions. Just as alcoholics are still responsible when they drink and drive, so too are internet addicts when they text or browse the web while driving. What's more, not all forms of distracted driving stem from internet addiction or, as we'll soon discuss, technology at all.

<u>Crack Down on Distracted Driving and Technology</u>

Texting while driving has become the poster child for distracted driving in the United States. According to the National Conference of State Legislatures (NCSL), texting while driving is banned in 47 states as well as all US territories. 14 of these states have taken the matter a step further and banned hand-held phone use completely. Some states have even banned cell phone use (hand-held or no) for certain demographics, like teen drivers.

The Problem of Enforcement

Of course, it's one thing to have these laws on the books and entirely another to adequately enforce them. Many of the laws are worded in such a way that they fall short of addressing the real problem. However, even if the laws are worded properly, it can be difficult for law enforcement officers to prove that drivers were indeed using their phones when they were driving. After all, there's no breathalyzer for texting.

First, let's examine the problem of wording. Many of the existing texting laws are very specifically about texting. However, smartphones have changed dramatically in recent years and drivers will use them for navigation, email, and even games. We know what you're thinking. The spirit of the law should cover all of these activities. Unfortunately, it's the letter of the law that matters in most courtrooms. Therefore, someone who was spending too much time looking at Google Maps and too little time looking at the road may get off on a technicality with nothing more than a slap on the wrist and a raised eyebrow that says, "we both know you should be in more trouble than this."

Let's assume that the law is worded perfectly and covers all manner of smartphone activities. A police officer is cruising down the highway when he spots you with a phone in hand. You're pushing buttons, glancing up every few seconds to make sure you're not in imminent danger of crashing into the car ahead of you. He slows to get behind you and flashes his lights. You slip the phone into your dash as you pull to the shoulder of the road. When the officer approaches your vehicle, he spots no smartphone. He only sees you with both hands on the wheel and an expression of wounded innocence. What is he supposed to say? That he swore you had a smartphone? Those proclamations don't tend to hold up in court.

Introducing the Textalyzer

These problems are not lost on police departments that are face with the impossible task of discouraging reckless driving habits. They also aren't lost on grieving parents like one Ben Lieberman whose 19-year-old son was killed when a distracted driver drifted into on-coming traffic and hit their car. The driver claimed that he had fallen asleep briefly when he drifted over the center lane and hit Lieberman's car head on. However, Lieberman suspected that the driver was actually texting.

Because cell phones are private property and contain private information, police officers can't access them without a warrant. With no probable cause to suggest that the driver was lying about his fatigued state, they had no means of getting one. Lieberman took matters into his own hands. Six months and one phone record subpoena later, he was able to show that the driver was lying.

Now, Lieberman wants to prevent other individuals from struggling as he did to find justice for themselves or loved ones. He co-founded an anti-texting advocacy group called Distracted Operators Risk Casualties (DORCS). Together with a tech company called Cellebrite, DORCS is creating a tool that will act as a breathalyzer for people's phones.

The technology would require a police officer to attach a cord to the driver's phone. This can be done right on the side of the road and while the phone is in the driver's possession. In other words, drivers do not have to surrender their phones to law enforcement. The device would then notify the officer of the last few actions taken on the phone along with a time stamp for each action. In this way, officers can determine with ease whether drivers were using their cell phones without needing a warrant for phone records. They'll also be able to tell if driver's were performing actions that wouldn't show up on a phone record, like accessing a website or sending an email.

Sounds simple, right? Truthfully, the technology has been met with some criticism. While it seems like an effective solution for the problem, it comes with its own complications. Phones and phone records require warrants for a reason. They are private property. Under this system, officers would be able to access the most recent phone activity based on little more than suspicion.

This has some privacy advocates crying foul and wondering if there isn't a better solution.

It's possible that with some regulation the technology could prove useful. Some proponents of the technology suggest only using it when there is a car accident and not during a traffic stop. Others wonder if the tech could be doctored so that it only shows time stamps for activity and not details about the nature of the activity. What's clear for now is that people have acknowledged the problem of enforcing texting laws and some big brains are getting closer to some viable solutions.

New Developments in Navigation Systems

While DORC and Cellebrite are working on the textalyzer, other tech companies have been puzzling out new ways to discourage people from using their phones on the road. Campaigns like "It Can Wait" emphasize the fact that some phone activities just flat out don't need to be performed in a moving vehicle. Missed calls, texts, and emails can all wait the fifteen minutes it will take to get home (or the five minutes it will take to find a parking lot). However, there is another phone function that is far more tempting for the average driver.

GPS navigation is more than just a luxury at this point. Many people use it daily to get from one location to another. Many millennials even admit to using it when they already know how to get some place purely to determine the fastest route and avoid high traffic. More and more cars come equipped with GPS ready technology, including displays that hang out above the radio and show the suggested route. For those who don't have the benefit of a display, there are dashboard holsters for cell phones that act as makeshift displays.

However, these tools have themselves shown to be distracting and dangerous. After all, they draw the eyes away from the road, requiring drivers to glance occasionally down in order to make sure they are still on track. Unfortunately, without a passenger to call out directions and assure the driver that he or she is on track, there's little that a driver can do.

<u>Managing Backseat Drivers</u>

Leaving aside technology for the moment, let's explore some of the other common distractions that face drivers. Although it may not seem it, side seat and backseat drivers can be as harmful to your driving concentration as a GPS screen or cell phone – and not necessarily in the ways you'd think. Backseat driving can be distracting and alarming (particularly if the person is trying to micromanage a left turn or chronically afraid of every other vehicle on the road). It can also be infuriating and that frustration you feel can negatively impact your driving long after the backseat driver has backed down.

Why We Backseat Drive

The term is often applied to any situation where a passenger in a car suggests an action or expresses anxiety over the driving. You may have heard yourself tell your significant other to stop being such a backseat driver when he or she suggested you avoid the highway during rush hour. However, true backseat driving, the kind that can impair the driver, is incessant and often unreasonable.

People who fall into this pattern might do so because they don't trust the driver's skill (as with a parent and a teenager). It's also possible they are just a nervous passenger, having been in a car accident. They may not like having other people control their vehicle and only engage in the behavior when a passenger in their own car. Whatever the reason, it's important to understand it if you're going to productively manage a backseat driver and diffuse a tense situation.

Strategies for Handling Backseat Drivers

- **Plan ahead.** Many backseat drivers are overly concerned with directions and the chosen route. If you're planning a longer trip with a friend that you know will likely give you a hard time, make the route decisions beforehand. Of course, this may not stop them from offering up their opinion mid drive anyway, but if will reduce the likelihood.

- **Use GPS.** Along these same lines, use GPS to choose the best route for you. After all, GPS has technology that you and your backseat driver don't. Who can argue with that?

- **Take breaks.** Backseat driving can become worse when people are tired, uncomfortable, or frustrated. Take frequent breaks on long trips to improve everyone's mood and reduce this effect.

- **Assign them a task.** If you're backseat driver is tenacious, you may need to get a little more proactive. Ask them to do something for you that will distract them from the job of backseat driving. You might ask them to look up information on their smartphone about the place you're going to. You could also try to play a road trip game with them (one that's not too distracting for you of course).

- **Turn on the radio.** Are they still talking? Drown them out with some sweet oldies or a favorite talk radio station. This will be entertaining for both of you, and since boredom can lead to backseat driving, it'll help keep your passenger occupied. If it doesn't work, and your backseat driver is still at it, at least you have something to focus on that isn't their incessant nagging.

- **Acknowledge the problem.** Still no luck. It's time to get real. Explain to them that what they are doing is frustrating and distracting. Ask them to stop. Believe it or not, this can really work. Many backseat drivers don't realize that they are nagging and will make efforts to stop if it's pointed out to them. Of course, some might just get angry with you.

- **Offer them the wheel.** You can always pull a switcheroo and invite them to drive. For longer trips, you can suggest that the two of you trade off driving duties (something that you should be doing anyway). For shorter trips, you can simply say "why don't you drive this time and I'll drive tomorrow." Either they'll take the hint and shut up or take you up on your offer and you can show them what a polite passenger sounds like.

- **Get introspective.** Are you having a serious problem with backseat drivers? Is it not just one person but several? Do these people give each other as hard a time as they give you? You might consider the fact that you're not a very good driver and you are putting people on edge. If your backseat driver complains constantly about you breaking too hard at stop lights, don't write them off just yet. Instead, try breaking more softly.

You've pulled out all the stops and your backseat drivers are still giving you a hard time? There's nothing wrong with telling a troublesome passenger that you don't want to drive them anymore. It should be clear by now that distracted driving is a very real concern and could be dangerous for everyone in your car.

Managing Children in the Car

Imagine driving 70mph down the highway while your seven-year-old is throwing a tantrum in the back seat. He's tall and his legs can easily reach the back of your chair from his car seat. You know because he hasn't stopped kicking you for a half a dozen exits. Children may not be backseat drivers, but they can certainly cause a raucous.

We're not just talking about when your kid is having a meltdown either. Everything from being handed an empty snack wrapper to adjusting your rearview mirror for a better look at the little ones can impede your driving. Kids can cover windows, cause spills, and make loud and sudden noises. These distractions reduce visibility for the driver or even cause drivers to take their eyes off the road for precious seconds.

Distracted driving is a leading cause of accidents and kids present a constant and unavoidable distraction. Keep your family safe by cultivating car friendly kids who understand the importance of the driver's role in a moving vehicle.

Cultivate Car Friendly Kids

- **Have car rules.** If your child is old enough to follow rules, then it's time to make some special ones for the car. Kids are smart and they know that certain things that they can get away with at home, won't fly in other environments. It's time to stress the fact that the car is one of those environments where special rules need to be followed.

- **Follow through.** Don't just make rules; enforce them. Have real consequences when your kids behave inappropriately in your vehicle, even if that means pulling over or going home and missing out on an event or activity.

- **Have supplies ready.** Even short car rides can seem like years to small children. Have age appropriate toys and snacks within arm's reach. Make it so you're not riffling through your bag and so you never have to take your eyes off the road or both hands off the wheel.

- **Prioritize your driving.** Kids get upset. Babies cry. This can be difficult to deal with. Sometimes the parents of small children want nothing more than to reach back and let their infant know that they are right there. While it's natural and important to address the needs of upset children, it's not as important as safe driving. That might feel like a hard pill to swallow, but it's the truth. If you need to let your baby cry while you focus on finding a safe place to park, then do it.

- **Keep them in the back seat.** Car seats are legally required to be in the back seat anyway. However, if you have a nine-year-old that's big enough to be car seat free, you should still consider keeping him or her in the back. Rowdy children are mostly noise when they are behind you. But when they are next to you, the distraction factor multiplies by about a hundred. They can throw things at you, spill things on you, and mess with vehicle controls.

Developing Car Rules that Work

- **Emphasize safety.** Make sure your kids understand that the rules you set are to protect them.

- **Be consistent.** Don't slacken the rules. Keep them straight-forward and follow through.

- **Keep it simple.** You don't need to write them a manual. A handful of key car rules will be easier for all of you to remember.

- **Make it a joint effort.** Remind your kids that you need to follow car rules too. Talk about some of the things that you also do to be safe in the car.

When you're driving, your number one focus should always be the road. Stop allowing yourself to make excuses when it comes to checking a text, calling a friend, or leaning back to stop your son from drawing on the window. Sometimes it's easy to convince ourselves that certain things are too important to wait. What we should be asking ourselves is are those things more important than our lives.

The popular television show *Criminal Minds* did an episode where a disgruntled (and clearly mentally ill) driver took to shot gunning people on the road. It's that image of the furious highway bully with the trunk full of weapons that comes to mind for many people when they think of "road rage." In reality, road rage doesn't have to be nearly that dramatic, although it's no less dangerous. In fact, if you've ever white knuckled it behind the wheel of your SUV while shouting at someone who recently swung haphazardly into your lane, then you've probably felt a little road rage yourself.

Road Rage Stats

Gathering data on aggressive driving can be difficult. Typically, law enforcement will look at aggressive driving habits, but there's no way to know that aggressive drivers were experiencing road rage at the time of the incident. Often, the two get lumped together since road rage typically leads to aggressive driving habits.

However, as we detail in the next section, they are not exactly interchangeable.

Aggressive Driving and Deaths/Injuries

- 66% of traffic accidents that result in fatalities involve aggressive driving. (NHTSA)

- There were 292 fatalities as a result of aggressive driving in 2011. That number has risen to about 467 in 2016. (NHTSA)

- There were 620 road rage incidents involving guns in 2016. (The Trace)

Risk Factors for Road Rage

- Road rage is most common among males under 19 years of age. (NHTSA)

- Half of drivers who are subject to someone driving aggressively will themselves start driving aggressively. (NHTSA)

Number of Aggressive Drivers

- 2% of polled drivers admit to trying to run an aggressive driver off the road. (NHTSA)

- Nearly 80% of drivers experienced some form of anger or rage behind the wheel in 2016 (AAA)

- In 2016, about 8 million drivers in the United States acted on their road rage by engaging in aggressive behavior like ramming the back of another car or confronting another driver. (AAA)

- 51% of drivers polled admit to tailgating at some point in 2016. (AAA)

- 24% of drivers polled admit to trying to block another vehicle from changing lanes in 2016. (AAA)

- 4% of drivers polled admit to getting out of their vehicle to confront another driver in 2016. (AAA)

- 3% of drivers polled admit to bumping another vehicle on purpose in 2016. (AAA)

Road Rage vs. Aggressive Driving

You're driving home from a Friday night trip to the movies when a jaguar comes zipping by you at what has to be 95 miles per hour. It's weaving in and out of lanes, avoiding anyone who is going slower than it, which is just about everyone. When it comes up on a Toyota that's only going 80 in the fast lane, it creeps up a little too close for comfort. Is this road rage?

The National Highway Safety Administration would consider this aggressive driving, defining it as "the operation of a motor vehicle in a manner that endangers or is likely to endanger persons or property." People experiencing road rage are likely to drive in an aggressive manner. However, not everyone driving aggressively is doing so out of rage. They may just be impatient or naturally aggressive in their driving habits.

Although it isn't strictly road rage, aggressive driving deserves a mention in this chapter. It is far more common than all out road rage and is considered a factor in about two thirds of fatal accidents (note the statistic in the last section). Aggressive driving and road rage are often lumped together. However, it's important to understand what sets road rage apart and how to spot it on the highway. In the following sections, we talk about the tell-tale signs of both aggressive driving and road rage.

How to Spot an Aggressive Driver

Let's revisit that Jaguar for a moment. Imagine that you're in the Toyota. The Jaguar driver is so close behind you that you can clearly see the expression on his face. What's more, you can't see the front bumper of his car. It's almost impossible to believe that he hasn't already rear-ended you. At the earliest opportunity, he zips around you. Thank goodness you hadn't decided to change lanes at that point or you have collided. Before long, you're in his dust and you like it that way.

Truthfully, aggressive drivers are not all that difficult to spot. Although some can be more subtle than others, they all engage in similar behaviors as a result of their impatience and intolerance of other drivers.

- **Tailgating.** No, we're not talking about barbeques in the back of your pick-up outside of the local football stadium. When it comes to aggressive driving, tailgating refers to following another vehicle too closely. Tailgaters often follow vehicles so closely that they risk rear-ending either while driving or in the event of a sudden stop.

- **Erratic acceleration and breaking.** This is harder to spot when traffic is flowing smoothly. However, aggressive drivers are easy to spot on more congested roads. They'll be the ones accelerating rapidly and hitting the breaks hard. This behavior is illogical since said driver isn't getting home faster than anyone else. It also puts them (and those around them) at a high risk of fender benders.

- **Switching lanes quickly and without signaling.** This is another behavior that you're likely to see in denser traffic. Impatient highway drivers will try to weave through traffic with frequent lane changes. They'll do so quickly, often ignoring their turn signal. Like erratic breaking and acceleration, this behavior puts them at an increased risk of accidents. Depending on the speed of traffic, these accidents could be severe.

- **Speeding.** Ok, ok. We know that most drivers speed a little bit. Often the peed of traffic on a highway will be somewhere between 5 and 15 miles per hour above the limit. When we talk about speeding in this sense, we're really referring to excessive speeding – the kind that blow everyone else away.

- **Chasing the green.** You may not be familiar with this term, but you've definitely seen this in action. In Driver's Ed, we're taught that green lights mean "go," red lights mean "stop," and yellow lights mean "slow down." But some drivers seem to think yellow means "speed up" and will often coast through an intersection even seconds after a light turns red.

You in the Toyota did the right thing. You didn't panic. You didn't accelerate to unsafe speeds to accommodate the driver. You didn't honk or engage the driver in any way as he passed. Knowing how to conduct yourself when around aggressive drivers is an important part of avoiding accidents. Keep reading to learn more about what you can do to prevent disaster.

<u>How to Spot a Driver with Road Rage</u>

Road raged drivers will engage in most of the same behaviors as your standard aggressive driver. However, they may also do things to express their intense anger toward another driver. This is what sets them apart.

- **Flashing headlights.** Drivers will often flash their headlights to indicate their displeasure with another driver or to just plain irritate them. This is unsafe and distracting for everyone on the road.

- **Honking.** Sometimes this is the only time a driver can make him or herself heard. However, when used inappropriately, it can be distracting.

- **Obscene gestures or language.** Truly angry drivers will express themselves with verbal and physical cues through an open window. When drivers get to this point, it's best to ignore them and distance yourself.

- **Ramming or bumping.** Truly angry drivers could take things to the next level and attempt to "interact" with you with their vehicle. This is extremely dangerous. Thankfully, it's also unlikely to happen. However, as the stats above attest, it could be more common than you think.

Hard to believe that someone could act this way? Remember that road rage is not just anger or frustration. Psychologists suggest that those with road rage experience an extreme reaction to a lack of control. Pair this with the overwhelming sense that every event on the highway is a personal slight. Now you have someone with enough pent-up rage that they become capable of activities they'd never dream of doing in any other circumstance.

Road rage is dangerous and distracting to the enraged driver. However, it's equally dangerous to all the other drivers on the road. If you find yourself on the same stretch of highway as an enraged driver, it helps to have strategies in place for dealing with them.

<u>How to Manage Aggressive Driving and Road Rage</u>

If I was forced to cover the topic of aggressive driving and road rage by using only three words, I know exactly what those words would be – DO NOT ENGAGE! As the saying goes, it takes two to tango and it usually takes at least two people to escalate a situation.   If you don't not allow yourself to become part of the escalation process, it will be less likely that the incident will spin out of control. Of course, you'll sometimes get those extra aggressive drivers who are ready to jump out of their car with no provocation other than that they think you slighted them somehow. But in many cases, it only takes a little push from you to send someone on the edge into a frenzy. In other words, do your part to prevent aggressive driving and go out of your way to avoid confrontation.

- **Keep your cool.** Breathe. Remember that about half of drivers who are exposed to aggressive driving on the road will start driving aggressively. Break the cycle. More aggressive drivers on the road means more risk.

- **Do not react to the driver.** If the driver is shouting or making gestures, ignore it. Do not shout or gesture back. An enraged driver is not likely to be cowed by such an action.

It will only make a bad situation worse and may put you at greater risk.

- **Distance yourself.** If you are able to safely and legally distance yourself from the driver, then do so, even if it means slowing down to let the angry driver pass or turning off of your intended route.

- **Keep driving.** Do not pull over and exit your vehicle. Do not engage the driver in any way. If the driver is enraged, you are safer in your car. Slow down if you have to, but keep driving.

- **Avoid eye contact.** After experiencing some kind of conflict with another car, whether they were tailgating us or we accidentally cut them off, most of us have been tempted to peek over at the other car to get a look at the driver. Is the person very old? Very young? Very angry? Fight this urge. Chances are they are trying to get a peek at you too and eye contact can aggravate frustration and anger.

It can be particularly tempting to try and teach aggressive drivers a lesson by preventing them from merging into your lane or brake checking them when they are tailgating you. However, these behaviors are just as aggressive and will only put lives at risk.

Brake Checking is a Big No

In 2016, a dashcam video went viral on YouTube. It came from the dashboard of a truck on a two-lane stretch of highway. However, the truck wasn't the subject of the video. The subjects were two SUVs traveling in the next lane a little ahead of the truck. One of the SUVs was tailgating the other, following so closely that it was in danger of rear-ending the car ahead of it. The car in the lead decided to hit the brakes quickly but firmly – an act known as "brake checking."

Brake checking is a popular way to warn tailgaters that they are following too closely. However, the brake check in this video did more than warn the tailgater; it ran him off the road. In the video, the car can be seen swerving from side to side, having lost control, and eventually driving straight into the ditch that divides the highway. At one point, it looks like the car might hit another in the lane next to it, but luckily no other cars were involved in the accident.

If you've ever suffered a tailgater before, then part of you is probably thinking that the SUV got what it deserved. If it hadn't been following so closely, then it would have been able to stop in time. But it's worth noting that the brake checker did so with the understanding that the car behind it would struggle to stop in time. That is, after all, kind of the point. That irresponsible choice put both cars at risk as well as every car in the vicinity. It's just as dangerous and irresponsible as the decision to tailgate.

Investigators agree the viral video soon caught the attention of local police. The tailgater was easily identified and cited. However, police then went on to try to identify the vehicle that did the brake checking before driving off into the distance. It is unclear whether they've been successful up to this point.

Long story short, don't brake check other drivers, no matter how reckless they are being. The only thing you'll be proving is that you're just as reckless as they are. And no slowing to a stop to annoy the tailgater like the UK driver who stopped on a highway in 2015. The tailgater managed to safely stop behind him before being rear-ended by speeding traffic. The only appropriate response to a tailgater is to take your lumps and get out of the way.

When to Call the Police

Sometimes road rage does go far beyond aggressive driving. In July 2017, a Pennsylvania teenager was shot in the head by another driver who was frustrated by their mutual attempts to merge when two lanes were being reduced to one. The man in question turned himself in, and at the time of writing, is facing first degree murder charges.

Even more recently, a four-year-old boy from Cleveland, Ohio was shot in the head when an incensed driver opened fire on an SUV. The boy miraculously survived and a warrant is out for the enraged driver. What facilitated this event? The boy's mother honked at the suspect's car when he blocked a road for more than five minutes. He then followed her onto the highway to commit the act.

It's safe to say that road rage is about more than just tailgating and flipping the occasional bird. It can get serious and fast. To hear the Pennsylvania driver's friends tell it, he was not an angry man. They seemed shocked to hear that he had shot anyone at all and described him as "even-keeled." Road rage can affect anyone and the results can be disastrous.

It's important, therefore, to understand when it's ok to call the police. You don't want to get on the horn every time somebody cuts you off. But if you feel that your safety is genuinely threatened, then you shouldn't be afraid to call for help. The following behaviors are not guarantees that the driver is about to pull out a gun, but they are evidence that the driver is acting overly aggressive toward you and intends to endanger or harm you.

- **Rear-ending.** A driver that rear-ends you on purpose is a driver that has crossed a major line. Nobody should be using their vehicle as a weapon or intentionally making contact with other vehicles.

- **Intentional swerving.** The aggressive driver may drive up next to you in the adjoining lane and attempt to edge you off the road. Slow down to avoid them. Exit as soon as possible.

- **Stopping and exiting vehicle**. If you're in slow traffic or stopped yourself and a driver who was driving aggressively approaches you on foot, it's time to get help. If you can, drive away. If you can't, seek help from bystanders, roll up your windows, and lock your doors. In both cases, call the police. Never exit your vehicle or confront a driver.

- **Pulling up beside you and shouting.** This may not seem as extreme as the others on this list. However, it is still an overly aggressive act and a sign that the driver is targeting you. If you feel threatened by a driver behaving in this way, roll up your windows and call for help. At best this is harassment, which is a punishable offense.

At the end of the day, be cool. It often takes two to tango. If you avoid shouting and honking at other drivers, you'll be less likely to get their blood up. Focus on getting where you need to go and don't worry about that driver that just pulled the illegal U-turn.

<u>Keeping Your Cool Behind the Wheel</u>

If you've ever heard someone tell you to "let it go," then you know how infuriating that phrase can be. When you're in the grips of anger, "letting it go" seems downright impossible. But sometimes all you need to do is take a few deep breaths or eat a favorite snack to feel that anger pass away. If you struggle with anger while driving, work on finding a strategy that suits you. Use the following as a starting point.

- **Breathe** – Always try this first. You can do it right away in your car without having to pull over. Take a single deep breath. Then another. Not in the mood to breathe? You don't have to be. Just force yourself to go through the motions. Breathing deeply and slowly can induce relaxation and reduce anger. The more you make a habit of trying this, the more likely you are to commit to it each time.

- **Stretch** – Ok. This one is a little trickier when you're in a moving vehicle. If you can't stop, try simply sitting up straight and stretching your spine. You can also roll your shoulders and your head (a little bit) without taking your hands off the wheel or your eyes off the road. If you can pull over and take five, try stretching a little more deeply. Focus on your arms, shoulders, and neck. This is where stress tension tends to collect.

- **Turn on some music.** – Well, this depends a little on you and a lot on the type of music you enjoy listening to. If you're likely to turn on heart-pounding rock, then maybe pass on this strategy. However, if you know any easy listening stations, some music could be a calming influence. Not to mention, just changing things up a little in the car might help snap you out of your bad mood.

- **Turn down your music.** – Maybe you already had some music on. Maybe you were rocking out to some old school

ACDC when you were cut off for the third time that day. Blasting Hells Bells is probably not the best way to keep yourself from flying into a rage. Dial it back a notch or three and consider switching to a smoother station (or switching it off).

- **Switch to talk radio.** – Talk radio may not be particularly calming, but it is certainly distracting. Get your mind onto a different subject by tuning into NPR or a comedy station.

- **Slow down.** – Literally, slow down. Angry people tend to drive more quickly. Focus on your speed and tap on the breaks. This will prevent you from driving at an unsafe speed and it may also have a calming effect.

- **Phone a friend.** – Only do this if you have a car phone or hands-free device. Talking to a friend, but not about what just happened. That'll only make you angrier. Ask them to tell you about their day or tell them about something good that happened to you.

- **Exit the highway.** – If you're on the highway and you can do so safely, get off of it. Driving on less busy roads, and ones with lower speed limits, ma have a calming effect on your nerves. Plus, it's safer for you to take some time away from the freeway.

- **Pull over.** – If possible (and again, if you can do so safely), pull over and stop your vehicle. This is an extreme strategy, but it's worth considering if you think your anger could be affecting your driving. Your safety and the safety of everyone else on the road is of the highest importance.

While these strategies will get you started down a path to more relaxed driving, they are only short-term solutions. If you find yourself needing to phone a friend or breathe slowly every other time you get behind the wheel, then you should look deeper.

What Makes an Aggressive Driver?

It may be hard for the cool-headed drivers out there to believe, but aggressive drivers are not simply aggressive and mal-adjusted people. Some generally level-headed and reasonable individuals can transform into angry and frustrated drivers at the drop of a hat.

The famously bitter comedian Luis C.K. acknowledged his own struggles with angry driving in a popular stand-up bit. He describes how bizarre it is that he, and many others, feel so comfortable yelling expletives at others on the road when we would never dare to do the same in other situations. Imagine shouting at a driver to get out of the way (possibly with some more choice words involved). Luis C.K. asks if you would say the same type of thing to someone on an elevator. What about in line at a coffee shop?

Comedians are not the only ones to notice this phenomenon. An animated short from the 1950s featuring the lovable Disney dog Goofy told the story of Mr. Walker. Mr. Walker was a model citizen until he got behind the wheel of his car. Like Jekyll into

Hyde, Walker transforms physically and emotionally into Mr. Wheeler. This not so model driver yells at others on the road and flies into uncontrollable fits of rage. Was Disney telling modern rendition of the famous Shelley horror story with their film *Motor Mania*? Maybe. It's more likely that they were holding up a mirror for the rest of us to get a good hard look at who we really are when we think we're being a good driver.

Something about being behind the wheel of a car makes us feel immune to the social norms that typically hold us back. That's not to say that we are all secretly ticking time bombs of rage, but that when our inhibitions are released, we are less likely to keep our anger in check. And anger can spiral out of control with alarming ease.

Psychologists call this mentality "deindividuation." In other words, when a person is in a large group, he or she loses her sense of individuality. This is not exclusive to driving. It's this loss of self-awareness that leads to things like "group think" where individuals tend to go along with a group instead of making their own decisions. The biggest problem with deindividuation is that it causes people to forgo any sense of personal responsibility. Add to this the relative anonymity that the road provides, and you've got a recipe for one pissed off driver.

It Can Wait

No, we're not talking about the popular texting and driving social awareness campaign. We're talking about your job, your date, or whatever else it is that you're in such a hurry to get to. Because isn't that really what all this aggressive driving comes down to? Your needs are more important than those of other people on the road. Your appointments are more pressing. You can't let that person merge because you have places to be, but you're angry at the person who won't let you merge because, well, you have places to be.

In many ways, an aggressive driver is a selfish driver. If you find yourself struggling with anger behind the wheel, then try to exercise a little empathy for your fellow drivers. Remember that the person trying to merge in front of you may have something important to get to as well. Of course, they may not, but that's not up to you to know or judge. Fight deindividuation and remind yourself constantly that every person on the road is an individual with their own story behind their driving habits. More importantly, remind yourself that you too are an individual and solely responsible for your actions on the road.

Finally, no place or appointment is more important than your life or the lives of others on the road. If you feel your anger rising in your throat, remember that being late is not the end of the world. Embrace the possibility of lateness and enjoy the ride.

<u>Stress and Your Health</u>

A single incident of road rage is not likely to have significant negative impacts on your health. However, if you make it a habit to lose your cool, then the constant stressors may have long term consequences. Every emotional reaction is also a physical one. And while you may feel relaxed after your anger passes, your body is still dealing with the fallout.

The Fight or Flight Response

Periods of extreme anger activate what is commonly referred to as the "fight or flight response." In other words, our bodies go into emergency mode. Our adrenaline (epinephrine) and cortisol levels skyrocket, leaving us with a heightened sense of panic and awareness. Of course, we have these hormones for a reason. The fight or flight response is essential for helping us get out of real danger. But while a grizzly bear standing an uncomfortable distance away might constitute danger, zipping along the highway in our car does not.

What exactly do these hormones do? They increase our heart rate, blood pressure, and metabolism. They also make us breathe more heavily as our bodies prime themselves for a fast response. This is a good thing in an emergency. The rapid breathing gets more oxygen into our lungs, oxygen that is promptly pumped to our vital organs and, most importantly, our brain. The increased awareness is essential if we want to react quickly. Finally, our livers produce more sugar, giving us the energy to act quickly.

Why does out body react to extreme anger the same way it reacts to extreme danger? For one thing, the portion of our brain that is responsible for sending out these hormones (known as the amygdala) is also responsible for emotional processing. Therefore, emotions rather than logic are responsible for triggering the response. In fact, this relationship is so closely tied that the fight or flight response can be triggered by things as benign as extreme loneliness or pessimism. If we allow our anger to get out of control, then it can easily have the same result.

If your body is kicking into overdrive every other morning commute, then these stress hormones and the physical effects they bring about will wear on you over time.

- **Diabetes** – Remember how we said your liver would start producing more sugar? Well, that sugar has to go somewhere after the "threat" has passed. It gets reabsorbed into the body. However, continued overproduction of sugar can lead to complications in those predisposed to developing Type II diabetes. Individuals who are heavily overweight are also more susceptible.

- **Migraines** – When you're stressed, your muscles become tense. That's your body preparing itself for a fight (literally). However, continued tension of the shoulders, neck, and back due to repeated episodes of high stress can lead to chronic tension and migraine headaches. It may also lead to muscle problems in those areas.

- **Heart Diseases** – Continued episodes of rapid pulse and high blood pressure could lead to consistent high blood pressure (hypertension), which in turn could lead to a heart attack or stroke. For people who already suffer from high blood pressure, a moment of extreme anger may even be the immediate catalyst for a heart attack or stroke.

- **Ulcers** – Stomach ulcers, also known as gastric ulcers, are painful sores that develop in the stomach. These sores can be caused by increased stomach acid resulting from chronic stress. At best, ulcers are nuisances that cause a burning pain in the stomach. At worst, they can grow large enough to perforate the wall of your stomach, allowing stomach acid to pass through and into your abdomen. This is life-threatening and requires immediate medical attention. If you already have an ulcer, then periods of extreme stress will make it worse.

- **Irritable Bowel Syndrome** – This mystery condition has no clear causes, but it has been heavily linked to chronic and severe stress. Stress can also make the symptoms worse for those who already suffer from the disease. Symptoms vary widely in severity and range from gas and bloating to severe abdominal pain.

- **Decreased testosterone** – This is obviously specific to men. Chronic episodes of stress can negatively impact testosterone production, which in turn affects sperm count and can lead to erectile dysfunction. Increased cortisol levels lead to lack of sleep, which in turn leads to even more cortisol. This poor sleep has an almost instantaneous effect on testosterone.

- **More painful periods** – Women aren't immune to gender specific effects. Chronic stress and increased stress hormones can lead to hormonal fluctuations that affect that time of the month. The result can be longer, more painful periods and more severe Premenstrual Syndrome (PMS) symptoms.

Think we're blowing a lot of smoke? Researchers like Laura Kubzansky, an assistant professor at the Harvard School of Public Health, have tracked the relationship between bouts of extreme rage and Coronary Artery Disease (CAD). Kubzansky notes that research strongly supports a correlative relationship between CAD and unchecked anger. With reports like *Angry Drivers Have Higher Risk of Collision* in Science Daily telling us that our lives are threatened every day by aggressive driving habits, it would seem that there's no escaping the consequences of our own angry driving, whether immediate or long term.

Let's start with an attitude check. You're probably prepared to skip this chapter. It's been a while since you've been in Driver's Ed, but you remember the important points. After all, you've been driving for years – you're practically an expert. That attitude is a big part of the problem. The more confident you are in your driving skills, the more likely you are to break certain rules because, well, you know you can handle it.

Don't Weave

The highway weaver is the perfect example of this. They zip in and out of lanes with seeming grace, convinced that their superior driving skills make them capable of avoiding collisions and anticipating other drivers' moves. The truth is, while you feel capable of avoiding other drivers, they may not be able to avoid you (or other cars).

Picture this. You are in the far left lane and coming up on the car in front of you. You're going 80 and they are only going 75. You spot a gap between them and the car in the lane to your right. If you come up from behind and slip in front of the right lane car, you won't have to reduce your speed. You pop on the blinker for a few clicks and make your move.

Now imagine you're the car in the right lane. You want to get into the left lane but only after you pass the car to your left – the one going 75. You press on the gas and slowly start to speed up. Suddenly there's a car in front of you and you have to swerve into the lane to your right to avoid rear-ending it. That the car had its blinker on is irrelevant because it came from behind. You wouldn't have been able to see it anyway.

What's the problem with this picture? It starts with the highway weaver.

- **The blinker.** You used the blinker without any consideration for what it might actually be for. You didn't think that the car that really needed to be notified of your merge had no way of seeing your blinker. Never merge from behind.

- **The assumptions.** Had the car in the right lane maintained its speed, you would probably have been fine and not caused the car to swerve or brake. But why would it necessarily do that? Highway weavers have a habit of assuming that every other car will continue to behave in the same way it has been behaving. They have a habit of seeing themselves as the only individual on the road and everyone else as a prop.

- **The impatience.** Finally, does it really matter that you get in front of the other car that quickly? How much will this move really gain you and at what cost? Unless you're a

Formula 1 or Nascar driver, then driving should never be a race.

There is a small chance that if you weave like this you might get where you're going faster. However, heavy traffic is heavy for everyone. There's an even better chance that the weaver that just zipped past on your left isn't going very far. Soon you'll be trundling past him as he's stuck behind a wall of vehicles in the other lane.

<u>Practice Defensive Driving</u>

People who tend to drive aggressively sometimes turn their nose up at the very concept of defensive driving. They erroneously assume that a good driver is a smooth risktaker – in other words, someone who is confident and assertive on the road. However, defensive drivers are good drivers because they understand how to read situations in a way that promotes everyone's safety.

Defensive Driving and the Overly Cautious

Part of the reason for this negative view of defensive drivers is the overall impression that defensive drivers are meek and uncertain. Some people envision elderly people who keep their blinker on for several blocks or a soccer mom who refuses to make left turns. These people are not driving defensively so much as overly cautiously. The former is a sign of a good driver, the latter is anything but.

The truth is that driving too cautiously can present its own problems on the road. Refusing to take a right on red when it is acceptable to do so can hold up traffic and frustrate other drivers. So too can waiting for a gap that you could land a jet in whenever you're turning onto a busy road. Sometimes driving too cautiously can even earn you a traffic ticket, as in cases where there is a minimum speed posted and you're trundling along five miles per hour below it.

If you can believe it, being overly cautious may even result in accidents. Of course, these accidents are more likely to be fender benders than they are to be multi-car pileups. However, they are accidents nonetheless. Like aggressive drivers, overly cautious drivers can be unpredictable. A predictable and skilled driver adheres to the rules and norms of the road. An overly cautious driver second guesses him or herself at every turn. They ignore certain road norms (as described above) and handle others poorly as they question their decisions. Overly cautious drivers are also more likely to hit their breaks without warning.

Given this behavior, it's no wonder that many people have such negative associations with defensive driving. However, it's important to understand that a defensive driver is not an uncertain one. A defensive driver knows and adheres to the laws and norms of the road. They just do so with a careful eye on everyone else.

But What Does That Mean?

It's all well and good to say that a defensive driver is aware of the other cars on the road, but how do they manage to be so aware? What does defensive driving look like? [possibly beef up intro]

Expect the unexpected. This is the number one skill of the defensive driver. Remember the scenario with the highway weaver? Defensive drivers behave in an opposite manner. They never assume that other cars on the road are going to maintain their behavior. In fact, they expect that many cars are going to behave dangerously. A defensive driver would see that highway weaver approaching in the rear-view mirror and slow down to let him or her merge safely. The following are some other ways that defensive drivers can anticipate problems on the road.

- Wait a beat when the light turns green to avoid colliding with anyone on the opposite road who might have been racing to beat their red light.

- Maintain a safe following distance in case the car in front of you breaks unexpectedly.

- In poor weather, assume that other cars might have problems with ice and visibility.

- Keep an eye on cars in highway lanes adjacent to yours. Watch for blinkers and drifters.

- Always check your blind spot before merging.

- Be mindful of highway exits (and who might be trying to get on and off).

In addition to anticipating problems, defensive drivers are alert and reactive. They know all of the rules of the road and follow them. At the same time, they don't expect that everyone else will know or follow the same rules.

The Benefits of a Defensive Driving Course

If you want to learn more about defensive driving, you should look into a defensive driving course. Look for certified course offerings on the website for your local DMV. While it's a good idea to take one of these courses just so you can become a better driver, these courses also offer benefits for people who've had some problems on the road. Exactly how a defensive driving course can help you may depend on your county, state, or auto insurance company. The following examples come from the Colorado DMV website.

- Get a traffic ticket dismissed.

- Prevent points from being added to your license or remove ones from your license.

- Avoid rate increases on your auto insurance policy.

- Get a "safe driving discount" with your auto insurance company.

The American National Standard for *Safe Practices for Motor Vehicle Operations* defines defensive driving as "driving to save lives, time, and money, in spite of the conditions around you and the actions of others." Yes, that means submitting to an aggressive driver instead of racing them, blocking them, or trying to teach them a lesson. Yes, it means putting others before you. And yes, it means having your priorities straight.

Minimum Safe Distance

While talking about defensive driving, we mentioned minimum safe distance. Let's take some time to explore this more, what it really means to be a safe distance away, and why this is so important. Different people define "minimum safe driving distance," well, differently. There are a variety of tips and general "rules of thumb" that have been touted over the years, and not all of them are precisely the same. We've covered the two most popular rules below.

The Car Length Rule

Many people will tell you that you should have the length of two cars between you and the car ahead of you. Anything less than this is considered tailgating. However, there are some flaws with this rule. Firstly, what kind of car are we talking about? If you're driving an SUV and the car ahead of you is a VW Bug, are you staying two SUV lengths away or two VW lengths away?

Let's assume it's the former (that would make the most sense given the lengthier breaking distance that a larger vehicle would have). How exactly are you supposed to eyeball it? This well-intentioned rule of thumb doesn't exactly tell you how to estimate a safe distance from within your vehicle.

Finally, this rule doesn't take speed into account. It will not take a heavy pick-up truck traveling 80mph the same amount of distance to stop as the same truck traveling 40mph. At what point is two whole vehicle lengths not enough?

Two-Second Rule.

This rule of thumb is a little easier to follow. It dictates that you should remain roughly two seconds behind the vehicle in front of you. Pick a landmark as you're driving, like a fire hydrant or street sign. Start counting when the car in front of you passes it (i.e. the back of the car is level with the object) and stop when you reach it (i.e. the front of your car is level with the object).

The two-second rule is popular because it is applicable to any speed. It doesn't run into the same problems as the car length rule. The amount of distance between the two cars will vary depending on the speed at which those cars are traveling. In fact, the two-second rule is roughly equivalent to a car's length for every 5mph of speed. Using this rule, two cars traveling 50 miles per hour should be about ten cars apart.

The most common criticism of the two-second rule is that everyone counts two seconds differently. Is it two quick seconds? Two "mississippis"? Thankfully, there's a solution to this conundrum. It is commonly suggested that instead of counting to two, drivers utter the phrase "only a fool breaks the two-second rule." Just don't talk too fast.

What exactly is the big deal about maintaining a safe distance? You've been driving for decades and you've never encountered a scenario where you couldn't break in time or had to swerve onto the shoulder of the road. Isn't it enough to just be able to see the road in front of you?

Driving rules are not for everyday drama. They are for those rare moments when things go wrong. Adhering to these rules could be the difference between life and death. Unless you possess a sixth sense that tells you when things are about to go wrong, then you need to practice smart defensive driving at all times.

Think of it as an insurance policy. Maintaining a minimum safe distance between you and the car in front of you gives you an escape route when accidents happen. In this way, when there's a bad accident and a multi-car pile-up, yours doesn't become the top car on the pile.

Know Your Car

Not all cars are created equal. Some are big and take a while to stop. Some have overly sensitive brakes. Some handle fine on a perfect day but fall apart the minute it starts to rain. Your car's weight, age, brakes, and tires all factor in when you brake. Therefore, a minimum safe distance for your car isn't necessarily the same for another. Know your car. Pay attention to how long it takes to brake. Be aware of how it handles in poor weather. Use your best judgement and always err on the side of more space.

When to Use Your Horn

People use their horns too much and, at the same time, not enough. Basically, you hear it plenty when drivers are frustrated or angry. It's the only sure-fire way that drivers have to tell others how they feel short of getting out of their car and banging on someone's windshield. But the horn was never intended as an honorary expletive or symbolic middle finger. What's worse, all of this horn misuse leads to more anger and more accidents. So, when is it a good time to use your horn?

- **Announce your presence.** Sometimes cars want to enter certain spaces and can't because your car is in the way. This happens when drivers almost back into you in a parking lot or try to merge into your lane without checking to see if you're there. Use your horn. It doesn't have to be a matter or frustration, although you may be feeling alarmed and frustrated. A quick clear note is all that's needed to tell a car "hey, I'm here."

- **Warn pedestrians.** Like cars, pedestrians sometimes make a move without looking where they are going. Jaywalkers may tear across the street or crosswalk pedestrians may get bored waiting for the walk signal. Whatever the reason, it's up to you to tell them that the way is not clear and you're in danger of hitting them.

- **Warn others of danger.** Sometimes drivers can see imminent accidents even when they aren't involved. You could be stopped at a stop light and notice that the driver coming up to your right is about to run the red. A quick honk on your horn will snap every driver to attention and could prevent a collision.

- **Notify others of traffic signals.** This has less to do with immediate safety and more to do with following traffic laws and not holding up traffic. Let's say someone is stopped at a light in front of you. The light turns green but the someone doesn't go. It's likely they are texting or looking at directions. Give them some time to react and then lightly tap the horn to get their attention. This is a safer and less confrontational action than getting out of your car to tell them to move.

Notice that horn usage is largely about alerting others to danger that you are aware of and they may not be. It can also be used to generally increase others' situational awareness. Its purpose is to promote safety and stability on the road. Of course, that's not how it is often used. There are plenty of times when horns are used irresponsibly.

- **Anger management.** If another driver's irresponsible behavior is about to land you both in an accident, go ahead and lay on the horn. However, if the threat is past and you're just angry at the driver in front of you who cut you off, forget about it. The horn is not a tool for you to express your feelings.

- **Saying hello to friends.** Is that your pal from work walking his dog along the boulevard? You tap the horn to make him look up and, startled, he does. Sure, there's no real danger with this approach, but by using the horn too liberally you are desensitizing everyone's reaction to it. The more people hear horns, the less effective they will be.

- **Celebration.** Let's say you're driving down the freeway and listening to the big game in the car (read: whatever sport you like). Your team scores the winning touchdown, basket, goal, etc. You (and many before you) may be tempted to honk your horn in excitement. It's especially fun when multiple cars join in. Think again.

Sure, you're not really hurting anyone. But this kind of behavior desensitizes people to the true purpose of the horn. Do your part to keep the roads safe and save the honking for when it really matters.

<u>The Skinny on Speeding</u>

Speeding is a bit of a sensitive topic. Depending on who you ask, you should stay five miles below the limit, ride the limit, extend five miles above the limit, or forget about the limit and just ride with the flow of traffic. How are you supposed to conduct yourself appropriate on the highway with so many competing points of view?

Unfortunately, there is no right answer. How speeding is addressed depends on the road, the traffic, the weather, and even just the cops in that area. Even staying well below the speed limit, something you'd think would be a sure-fire way to avoid a ticket, can get you pulled over. Here are some tips for driving safely and with less risk of interference.

- **Pay attention to minimum speeds.** Some places have speed limits on both ends of the spectrum. Never dawdle below the lower limit unless you are forced to due to traffic. Keep an eye out for minimum speeds.

- **Go with the flow of traffic.** Basically, if you're above the speed limit, you don't want to look like you're speeding. In other words, if the speed limit is 65 and everyone in the left lane is going about 73, then don't start tailgating the person ahead of you. Stay with the crowd.

- **Only pass in the left lane.** This is sort of an extension of the last point. Being overly aggressive is not only unsafe – it also draws a lot of attention to your car. Cut out the weaving and drive responsibly (and inconspicuously).

Finally, whatever your speed, don't slam on the brakes when you see a cop car in the distance. This will put you and others at risk. What's more, if a police officer sees you do this, you might be in more hot water than if you'd just sailed on through.

Time to Get Real

Take a tour through the headlines in your local paper. Google "car accident" online and see how many news articles are from the past month, the past week, even the past day.

- A mother of 6 is killed by a drunk driver on her way to visit her premature twin girls in the neonatal unit of the local hospital.

- Two football players from Trinity Valley Community College are killed when their vehicle swerves into oncoming traffic at the ripe hour of 4am.

- A 69-year-old man dies in a crash involving multiple road raged drivers.

- A 33-year old man is charged with vehicular manslaughter after his drunk driving killed his infant daughter.

And this is only the tip of the iceberg. Driving is considered more dangerous, with more accidents and deaths per year, than flying. Think about that. When you get behind the wheel of a car to go to work, you are taking a greater risk than when you climb into a plane that soars thousands of feet into the air.

Driving is also more dangerous than skydiving. The likelihood of dying behind the wheel of a car is about 1 in every 6,000. For skydiving deaths it's 1 in every 100,000. That's right, literally jumping out of a plane with half a balloon strapped to your chest is statistically safer than going to work in the morning.

Why are we telling you this? Is it to convince you to skydive to work instead? No. We want you to think about why. After all, with so much experience driving, how is it that we can be so bad at it? One argument is that nobody is going skydiving without a boatload of precautions. The same can be said for pilots about to get in a cockpit. In other words, we recognize the dangers in these activities and we take them very seriously.

It's time we started taking driving more seriously.

Conclusion

As I put the finishing touches on this book, the calendar has turned to 2018. The passage of time, however, has not dulled my memories of Meghan. Not a day goes by when she is not in my thoughts. Sometimes I feel good reminiscing about the good times I shared with her, but at other times the pain of her loss still seems very fresh. Holidays are especially tough times of the year, as we just basically go through the motions with minimal acknowledgement of the day in my household. At least with holidays, the onset of depression is predictable. There are many other occasions when some completely random time and place will bring the emotions of losing Meghan rushing forth. It may be when I am driving past St. Gregory's, her grammar school, where I used to drop her off and pick her up each day. Sometimes emotions begin to churn when I pass the local park and see the swings and slides she used to play on. It could even be something as subtle as visiting the local Pizza Hut restaurant, where Meghan

and her brother Bryan used to love going to after school.

Another aspect of Meghan's loss that I would like to acknowledge

is the kindness of so many people towards my family and I.

Within these kind sentiments, however, was a well-meaning

statement that I heard regularly, that came close to making me

explode. I can't begin to explain the frustration of hearing over

and over again, "I know how you feel."   Anyone who has

experienced the tragedy of losing a child will understand my

point. Trust me – unless you have experienced the pain of losing

a child – you don't know how I feel. In 1982, my father died of a

sudden heart attack at the age of fifty-five. My dad was a vibrant

man who had not been significantly sick a day in his life. I was a

rookie cop on patrol at the time I was notified of his death. The

experience of losing my dad suddenly was devastating. As

horrible as my father's loss was, it was maybe 5% of the

devastation experienced at losing Meghan. The bottom line is losing a child is simply contrary to the laws of nature.

I haven't said very much about the man who killed my daughter. Frankly, there isn't much to say. He was found guilty of vehicular homicide and sentenced to 3.5 to 10 years in prison. In all likelihood he will be released from prison in 2019. Eight years was the legal value placed on Meghan's life. There is really nothing more to say.

I suppose the truly Christian thing to do would be to forgive this man who took Meghan's life with his selfish, criminal actions – but I can't. In all honesty, I wish him nothing but misfortune and misery for every day of the rest of his life.

The final message in this book is not to rant about the waste of humanity who killed Meghan. To the contrary, I assume that anyone taking the time to read a book on this important topic would find it impossible to do what he did. My closing message is simple. We all know what the right thing to do is, but we are all human beings, subject to the bad judgement inherent with being human. My plea goes out to good people who are in a situation where they are about to exercise bad judgement.

- You're leaving that party where you've had a couple of drinks. You feel ok, but as you slide into the driver's seat you know in your heart that you should not be driving.

- You've been battling a cough/cold, and the over the counter cough medicine you are using has helped, but it tends to make you drowsy after you take it. You just took some cough medicine and are now set to drive to work because you must attend an important meeting. As you back out of your driveway you know in your heart that you should not be driving after taking the cough medicine.

- You worked a double shift and when you got home you discovered that a pipe had burst in your basement. By the time the pipe was repaired and your basement was cleaned up, eight hours have gone by. You don't have to work today but you promised your mother, who lives forty miles away, that you would install an air conditioner in her bedroom window. You have not slept in 24-hours and as you begin the drive to your mother's house, you know in your heart that you should not be behind the wheel.

- You are driving on a two- lane road when a car accelerates past you at a high rate of speed and moves into your lane, cutting you off and forcing you to jam on the brakes. The vehicle that cut you off is now stopped at a red light and you have the opportunity to pull along-side. You are irate and you plan to roil down your window and express your displeasure verbally. As you roll down your window and prepare your first expletive, you know in your heart that you should not be engaging in this behavior.

If you experience any of these situations right after you finish this book or twenty years from now – please – think of my story and especially think of my Meghan. If only one person decides not to

drive after drinking, using medications, being overly tired, or

becoming angry on the road, then both you and I would have

honored the memory of Meghan. Be safe.

Bibliography

Aboujaoude, Elias, et al. "Potential Markers for Problematic Internet Use: A Telephone Survey of 2,513 Adults." CNS Spectrums, vol. 11, no. 10, 2006, pp. 750–755., doi:10.1017/s1092852900014875.

"Anaphylaxis." Mayo Clinic, Mayo Foundation for Medical Education and Research, 14 Feb. 2017, www.mayoclinic.org/diseases-conditions/anaphylaxis/symptoms-causes/syc-20351468.

Andrillon, Thomas, and Sid Kouider. "How your brain actually makes decisions while you sleep." The Washington Post, WP Company, 17 Sept. 2014, www.washingtonpost.com/posteverything/wp/2014/09/17/your-brain-actually-makes-decisions-while-you-sleep/?utm_campaign=pubexchange_article&utm_medium=referral&utm_source=huffingtonpost.com&utm_term=.f5f993004c26.

"Benzodiazepine Abuse." WebMD, WebMD, www.webmd.com/mental-health/addiction/benzodiazepine-abuse#1.

Brady, J. E., and G. Li. "Trends in Alcohol and Other Drugs Detected in Fatally Injured Drivers in the United States, 1999-2010." American Journal of Epidemiology, vol. 179, no. 6, 2014, pp. 692–699., doi:10.1093/aje/kwt327.

Brodwin, Erin. "What a legal drug that kills more Americans than heroin does to your body and brain." Business Insider, Business Insider, 11 May 2016, www.businessinsider.com/mental-physical-effects-of-opioids-2016-5.

"Colorado Amendment 64." Wikipedia, Wikimedia Foundation, 1 Nov. 2017, en.wikipedia.org/wiki/Colorado_Amendment_64.

"Colorado Defensive Driving & Traffic School." DMV.org, www.dmv.org/co-colorado/defensive-driving.php.

"Computer/Internet Addiction Symptoms, Causes and Effects." Signs and Symptoms of Internet or Computer Addiction, www.psychguides.com/guides/computerinternet-addiction-symptoms-causes-and-effects/.

Copeland, Larry. "Survey: Nearly a quarter of teens drive while impaired." USA Today, Gannett Satellite Information Network, 25 Apr. 2013, www.usatoday.com/story/news/nation/2013/04/25/teens-drunken-driving-impaired-survey/2106325/.

"Crime in the U.S. 2014." FBI, FBI, 19 May 2015, ucr.fbi.gov/crime-in-the-u.s/2014/crime-in-the-u.s.-2014.

"Defensive driving." Wikipedia, Wikimedia Foundation, 29 Aug. 2017, en.wikipedia.org/wiki/Defensive_driving.

"Defensive Driving 101." DMV.org, www.dmv.org/defensive-driving/defensive-driving-101.php.

"Driving under the influence." Wikipedia, Wikimedia Foundation, 6 Nov. 2017, en.wikipedia.org/wiki/Driving_under_the_influence.

"Drowsy Driving Statistics." Drowsy Driving Statistics - Sleep Education, school.sleepeducation.com/drowsydrivingstats.aspx.

"Drowsy Driving — 19 States and the District of Columbia, 2009–2010." Centers for Disease Control and Prevention, Centers for Disease Control and Prevention, 4 Jan. 2013, www.cdc.gov/mmwr/preview/mmwrhtml/mm6151a1.htm.

"Drunk Driving." NHTSA, 3 Nov. 2017, www.nhtsa.gov/risky-driving/drunk-driving.

"Epilepsy and Driving." Epilepsy and Driving | Michigan Medicine, www.uofmhealth.org/health-library/hw108709.

Fell, James. "Repeat DWI Offenders in the United States." NHTSA, NHTSA, 1995, one.nhtsa.gov/people/outreach/traftech/1995/TT085.htm.

"Field Sobriety Tests and Chemical Tests for DUI Defense." Lawfirms.com, www.lawfirms.com/resources/dui-and-dwi/dui-defendants-rights/field-sobriety.htm.

Gajewski, Misha. "Most sleep-Deprived nation? Study ranks Canada third out of 13." CTVNews, 28 Oct. 2016, www.ctvnews.ca/health/most-sleep-deprived-nation-study-ranks-canada-third-out-of-13-1.3136333.

Gardiner, Bryan. "Why Being on the Road Unlocks Our Worst Selves." Slate Magazine, 28 May 2015, www.slate.com/articles/health_and_science/science/2015/05/the_psychology_of_road_rage_driving_makes_you_angry_anonymous_and_emotionally.html.

"General Statistics and Facts about the Dangers of Drowsy Driving/ Fatigue." Stats: Drowsy Driving/ Fatigue, www.teendriversource.org/stats/support_teens/detail/65.

Gregoire, Carolyn. "5 Amazing Things Your Brain Does While You Sleep." The Huffington Post, TheHuffingtonPost.com, 28 Sept. 2014, www.huffingtonpost.com/2014/09/28/brain-sleep-n_5863736.html.

Hartman, R. L., and M. A. Huestis. "Cannabis Effects on Driving Skills." Clinical Chemistry, vol. 59, no. 3, July 2012, pp. 478–492., doi:10.1373/clinchem.2012.194381.

"Heart attack: Warning signs of a heart in trouble." Mayo Clinic, Mayo Foundation for Medical Education and Research, 29 July

2017, www.mayoclinic.org/diseases-conditions/heart-attack/basics/risk-factors/con-20019520.

"Heart attack: Warning signs of a heart in trouble." Mayo Clinic, Mayo Foundation for Medical Education and Research, 29 July 2017, www.mayoclinic.org/diseases-conditions/heart-attack/basics/symptoms/con-20019520.

"How Much Sleep Do We Really Need?" National Sleep Foundation, sleepfoundation.org/how-sleep-works/how-much-sleep-do-we-really-need.

"Hurricane Resources:" Stroke Warning Signs and Symptoms, www.strokeassociation.org/STROKEORG/WarningSigns/Stroke-Warning-Signs-and-Symptoms_UCM_308528_SubHomePage.jsp.

"Impaired Driving." Impaired Driving | AAA Foundation for Traffic Safety, www.aaafoundation.org/impaired-driving.

"Impaired Driving: MedlinePlus." MedlinePlus Trusted Health Information for You, medlineplus.gov/impaireddriving.html.

"Inducing Task-Relevant Responses to Speech in the Sleeping Brain." Current Biology, Cell Press, 11 Sept. 2014, www.sciencedirect.com/science/article/pii/S0960982214009944.

Jewett, Amy, et al. "Alcohol-Impaired Driving Among Adults — United States, 2012." MMWR. Morbidity and Mortality Weekly Report, vol. 64, no. 30, July 2015, pp. 814–817., doi:10.15585/mmwr.mm6430a2.

Jimison, Robert. "'Drugged driving' surpasses drunken driving in deadly crashes." CNN, Cable News Network, 28 Apr. 2017, www.cnn.com/2017/04/27/health/drugged-driving-death-rates-report/index.html.

Kam, Katherine. "Rein In the Rage: Anger and Heart Disease." WebMD, WebMD, www.webmd.com/heart-disease/features/rein-in-rage-anger-heart-disease#1.

Kaplan, Michael S. "Anaphylaxis." The Permanente Journal, vol. 11, no. 3, 2007, pp. 53–56., www.ncbi.nlm.nih.gov/pmc/articles/PMC3057722/.

"Lack of Sleep is Affecting Americans, Finds the National Sleep Foundation." National Sleep Foundation, sleepfoundation.org/media-center/press-release/lack-sleep-affecting-americans-finds-the-national-sleep-foundation.

Legal, Inc. US. "USLegal." Impaired Law and Legal Definition | USLegal, Inc., definitions.uslegal.com/i/impaired/.

Lewis, Kayleigh. "Adults in the UK are under-Sleeping by an hour every night." The Independent, Independent Digital News and Media, 1 Apr. 2016, www.independent.co.uk/life-style/health-and-families/health-news/adults-uk-under-sleeping-health-sleep-fatigue-a6963631.html.

McClurg, Lesley. "Is 'Internet Addiction' Real?" NPR, NPR, 18 May 2017, www.npr.org/sections/health-shots/2017/05/18/527799301/is-internet-addiction-real.

"NHTSA." NHTSA, 12 Sept. 2017, www.nhtsa.gov/.

Pack, Allan I., et al. "Characteristics of crashes attributed to the driver having fallen asleep." Accident Analysis & Prevention, vol. 27, no. 6, 1995, pp. 769–775., doi:10.1016/0001-4575(95)00034-8.

Paul, Jesse. "A month away from his Falcon High School graduation, teen is killed by suspected drunk driver." The Denver Post, The Denver Post, 17 Apr. 2017, www.denverpost.com/2017/04/17/falcon-high-school-teen-killed-crash/.

Pejovic, S., et al. "Effects of recovery sleep after one work week of mild sleep restriction on interleukin-6 and cortisol secretion and daytime sleepiness and performance." AJP: Endocrinology and Metabolism, vol. 305, no. 7, 2013, doi:10.1152/ajpendo.00301.2013.

"Police Department." Aggressive Driving, www.muni.org/Departments/police/traffic/Pages/AggressiveDriving.aspx.

SAMHSA, Center for Behavioral Health Statistics and Quality. "Results from the 2013 National Survey on Drug Use and Health: Summary of National Findings." Results from the 2013 NSDUH: Summary of National Findings, SAMHSA, CBHSQ, www.samhsa.gov/data/sites/default/files/NSDUHresultsPDFWHTML2013/Web/NSDUHresults2013.htm.

Schaper, David. "'Textalyzer' Aims To Curb Distracted Driving, But What About Privacy?" NPR, NPR, 27 Apr. 2017, www.npr.org/sections/alltechconsidered/2017/04/27/525729013/textalyzer-aims-to-curb-distracted-driving-but-what-about-privacy.

"Seizures: Causes, Symptoms and Diagnosis." Healthline, Healthline Media, www.healthline.com/symptom/seizures.

"Signs and Symptoms." Anaphylaxis Campaign, www.anaphylaxis.org.uk/hcp/what-is-anaphylaxis/signs-and-symptoms/.

Stafford, Tom. "Future - How sleep makes your mind more creative." BBC, BBC, 5 Dec. 2013, www.bbc.com/future/story/20131205-how-sleep-makes-you-more-creative.

"Texting While Driving in 2016." Texting While Driving in 2016 | CSG Knowledge Center, knowledgecenter.csg.org/kc/content/texting-while-driving-2016-0.

The Associated Press | Wire reports. "Breathalyzer for texting in works as road deaths on rise." MLive.com, MLive.com, 14 May 2017, www.mlive.com/news/us-world/index.ssf/2017/05/breathalyzer_for_texting_in_wo.html.

Walsh, J. Michael, et al. "Drug and alcohol use among drivers admitted to a Level-1 trauma center." Accident Analysis & Prevention, vol. 37, no. 5, 2005, pp. 894–901., doi:10.1016/j.aap.2005.04.013.

"Who Is at Risk for a Stroke?" National Heart Lung and Blood Institute, U.S. Department of Health and Human Services, 27 Jan. 2017, www.nhlbi.nih.gov/health/health-topics/topics/stroke/atrisk.

AP. "Why so many people text and drive, knowing dangers." CBS News, CBS Interactive, 5 Nov. 2014, www.cbsnews.com/news/why-so-many-people-text-and-drive-knowing-dangers/.

Wilson, Fernando A., et al. "Fatal Crashes from Drivers Testing Positive for Drugs in the U.S., 1993–2010." Public Health Reports, vol. 129, no. 4, 2014, pp. 342–350., doi:10.1177/003335491412900409.

"Woman caught on film 'using laptop at the wheel of Audi'." Evening Standard, 19 Apr. 2016, www.standard.co.uk/news/london/woman-caught-on-film-using-laptop-at-the-wheel-of-an-audi-while-driving-through-central-london-a3228721.html.

Young, Kimberly. "Internet addiction over the decade: a personal look back." World Psychiatry, vol. 9, no. 2, 2010, pp. 91–91., doi:10.1002/j.2051-5545.2010.tb00279.x.

About the Author

Robert L. Bryan was born in Queens, New York, and has been a life-long New York City resident. He retired after a twenty year career with the New York City Police Department at the rank of captain, and is currently the chief security officer at a New York State government agency. He is also an adjunct professor in the homeland security department of a NYC college. Robert has written several police related fiction and non-fiction books, as well as a non-fiction book regarding the profession of railroad conductor, inspired by his son's career. Two of his books – C-Case and Dark Knights – won awards at the 2017 Public Safety Writers Association writing competition. Impaired Driving/Shattered Lives is dedicated to his daughter Meghan, who was killed by an impaired driver in 2011.